THE PREGNANCY PRESCRIPTION

2nd Edition

An Essential Guide for
Understanding and Overcoming
Infertility

HUGH D. MELNICK, M.D., F.A.C.O.G.

DISCLAIMER

The information contained in this book represents the opinions of the author and should by no means be construed as a substitute for the advice of a qualified medical professional. The information contained in this book is for general reference and is intended to offer the user general information of interest. The information is not intended to replace or serve as a substitute for any medical or professional consultation or service. Certain content may represent the opinions of the Hugh Melnick, MD , based on his training, experience, and observations; other physicians may have differing opinions.

All information is provided "as is" and "as available" without warranties of any kind, expressed or implied, including accuracy, timeliness, and completeness. In no instance should a user attempt to diagnose a medical condition or determine appropriate treatment based on the information contained in this book. If you are experiencing any sort of medical problem or are considering cosmetic or reconstructive surgery, you should base any and all decisions only on the advice of your personal physician who examined you and entered into a physician-patient relationship with you.

ISBN-13 - 978-0-9792240-3-4
ISBN-10 -0-9792240-3-9

This book is designed to provide information of a general nature about medical procedures. The information is provided with the understanding that the author and publisher are not engaged in rendering any form of medical advice, professional services or recommendations. Any information contained herein should not be considered a substitute for medical advice provided person-to-person and/or in the context of a professional treatment relationship by a qualified physician, surgeon, dentist and/or other appropriate healthcare professional to address your individual medical needs. Your particular facts and circumstances will determine the treatment that is most appropriate to you. Consult your own physician and/or other appropriate healthcare professional on specific medical questions, including matters requiring diagnosis, treatment, therapy or medical attention. The information contained in this report is delivered "as is" without any form of warranty expressed or implied. Any use of the information contained within is solely at your own risk. MDPress, Inc. assumes no liability or responsibility for any claims, actions, or damages resulting from information provided in the context contained herein.

Printed in the United States of America.

Cover design by Jane Birkenstock
Book design by Jan Lakey

Photography of Dr. Melnick by Lou Manna

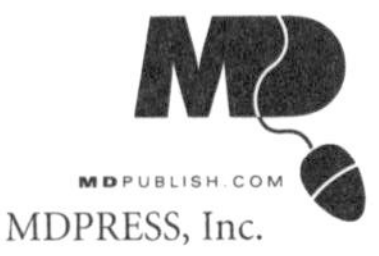

MDPRESS, Inc. 350 Fifth Avenue, Suite 7619-New York,NY 10118

ABOUT THE AUTHOR

Dr. Hugh D. Melnick is a graduate of the University of Pennsylvania and the Temple University School of Medicine. He was also a Research Fellow at the Queen Elizabeth Hospital in Birmingham, England. Completing his Post Graduate Training at Lenox Hill Hospital in 1976, Dr. Melnick has had over thirty years of clinical experience helping both couples and individuals who experience difficulty in becoming pregnant.

In 1983 Dr. Melnick founded Advanced Fertility Services, the first free-standing In Vitro Fertilization Center in New York City, where he has served as Medical Director since its inception. He is recognized as a pioneer in the development of outpatient IVF Clinics and is credited with successfully demonstrating that all types of fertility treatments can be provided safely and effectively outside of the traditional hospital setting. Most out-patient IVF Centers in the United States and abroad are based upon the Advanced Fertility Services model.

One of Dr. Melnick's most strongly held beliefs is that medical practice is an art that combines scientific knowledge, humanism and empathy. As such, the patients' emotional needs must be addressed at the same time that medical treatment is rendered. This is especially true when treating infertility since the inability to have a baby has a profound effect upon an individual's well-being as well as their relationship to their partner. Since conception normally takes some time to occur, Dr. Melnick believes that if a patient receives treatment in an emotionally supportive environment, they will be able to maintain the emotional strength needed to persevere until conception or resolution can occur.

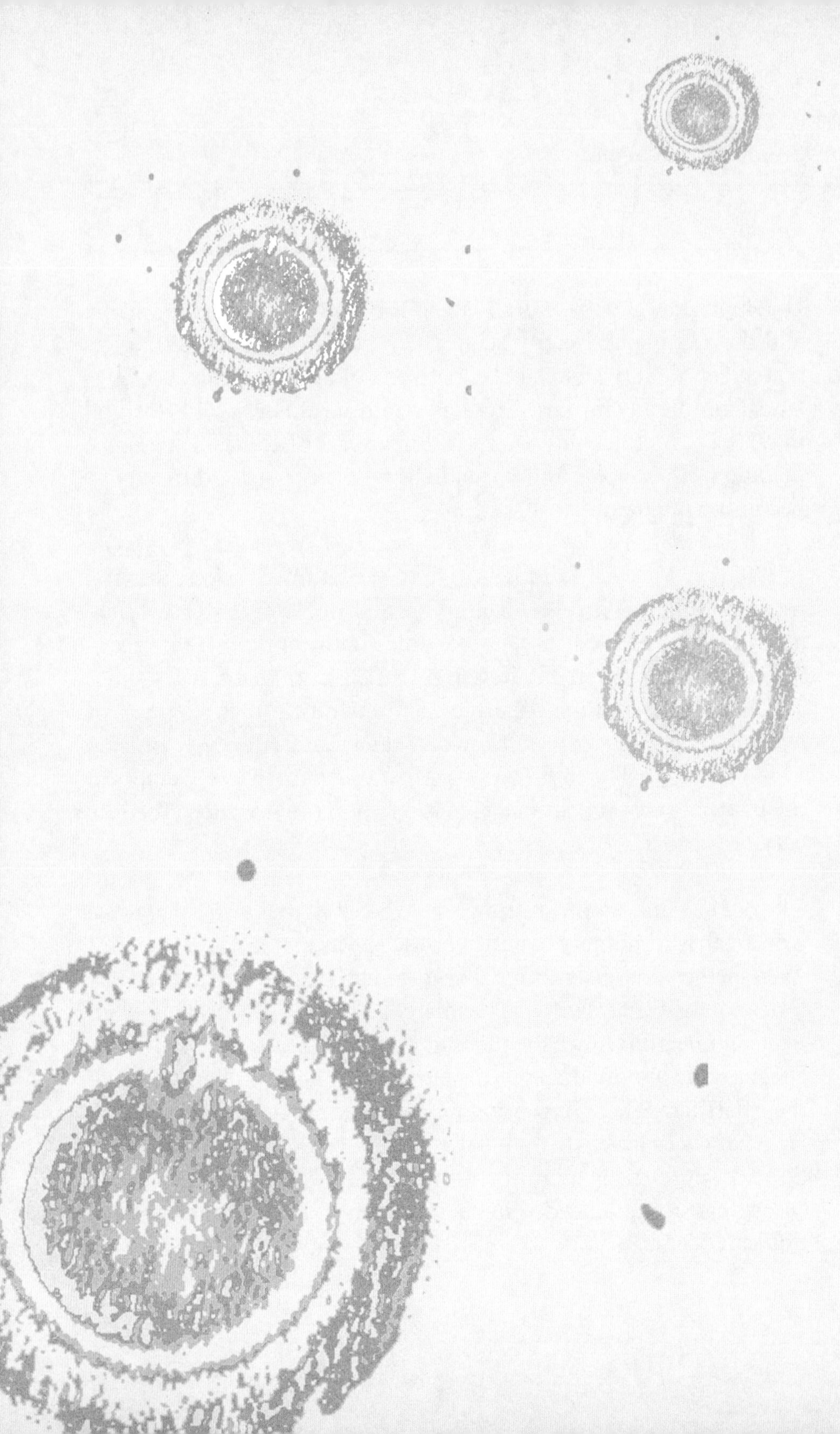

*To my beautiful wife, Lori–
you are the sunshine of my life. Thanks for lighting up my world with the sound of your joyous laughter and your radiant smile!*

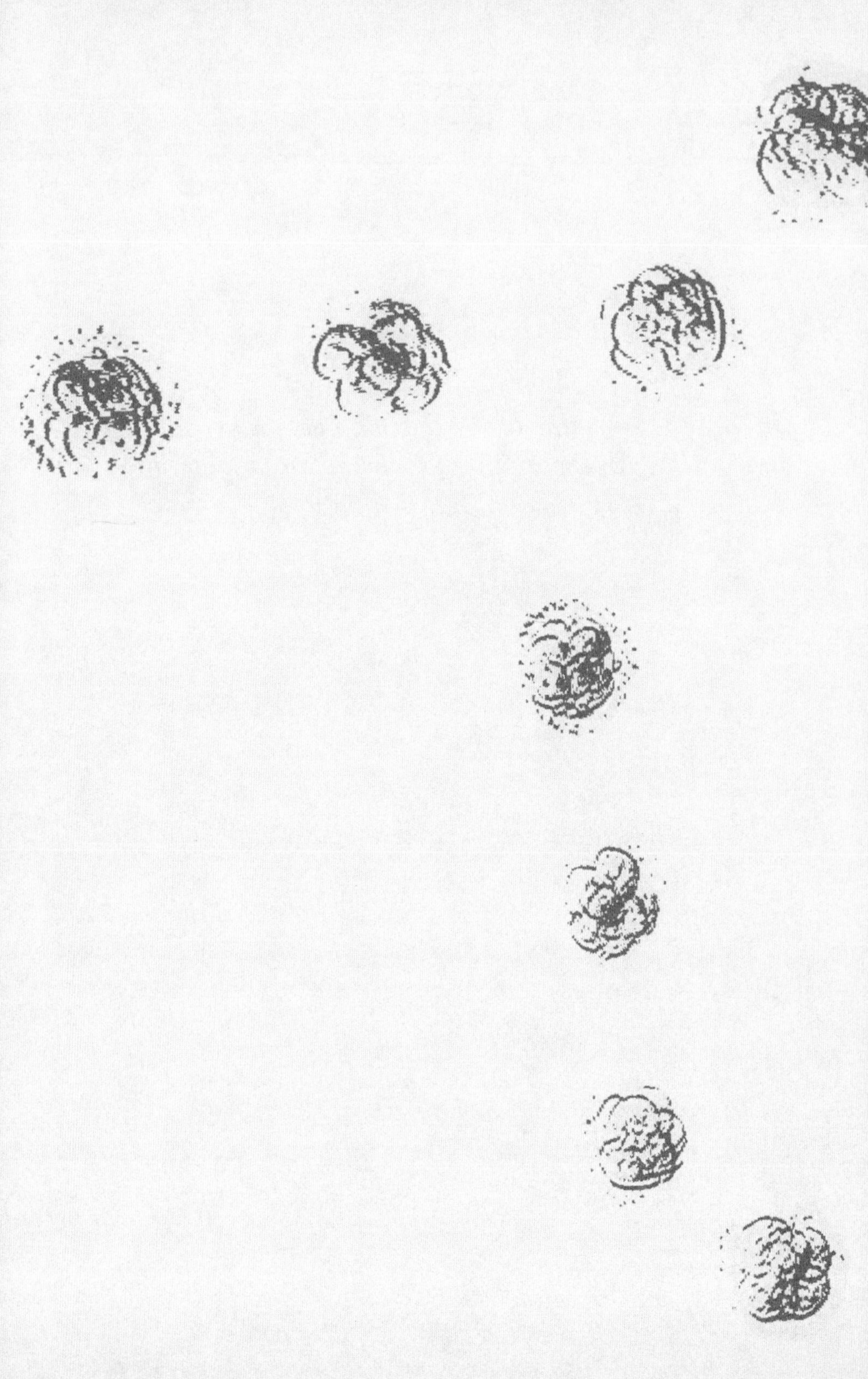

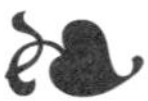

IN MEMORIAM

As I reflect upon my professional career, I give eternal thanks to those, no longer with me in the physical world, whose contributions have created the foundation that made it all possible. Nearly every day in my life, there is some instance in time that triggers fond memories of my parents, Everett and Selma, as well as my professional mentors, Hugh R.K. Barber, M.D. (Gynecological Surgery), Edward Graber, M.D. (Obstetrics and Gynecology), Herbert S. Kupperman, M.D., Ph.D. (Reproductive and General Endocrinology) and Herman Friedman, Ph.D. (Laboratory Science). Their teachings, guidance and example have served me well in my life. To honor their memories, my greatest hope is to pass on to others, in some way, the wonderful gifts that they have given to me.

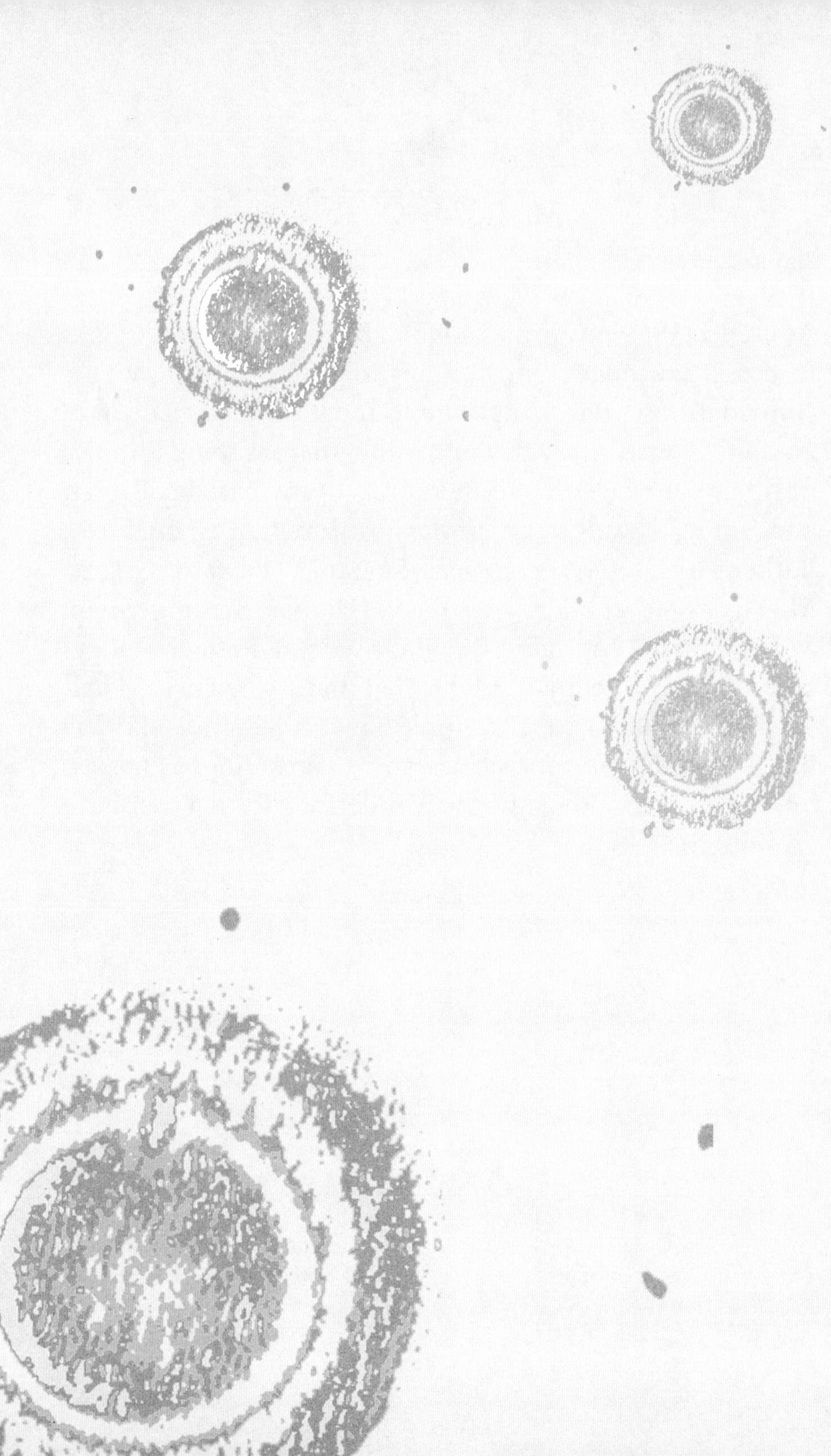

ACKNOWLEDGEMENTS

I would like to express my gratitude to Nancy Intrator, friend and "co-conspirator", who has made our collaboration on this book a truly joyous and intellectually stimulating experience. Her organizational genius has enabled me to mold thirty years of learning and experience into a cohesive story. I also wish to thank Luba Ruznikov, senior sonographer, *par excellance*, at Advanced Fertility Services, for not only the beautiful sonographic images appearing in this edition, but also for the many wonderful years that we have worked together. Luba has always been a great creative force in my professional life, for which I owe her a tremendous debt of gratitude. Many thanks also go to Kent Thanki, Ph.D., respected colleague of many years and the director of embryology at Advanced Fertility Services. His photographic images of eggs and embryos, the very earliest stages of human existence, provide a rarely seen view of the miracle of life. I also wish to thank Ms. Dana Alogna for her invaluable editorial assistance, as well as for the creation of all the graphics and the photographic layouts found in this edition. My gratitude also goes to Ms. Gilda Stahl, for all her editorial insights. Finally, I wish to thank all the wonderful people who make up the staff of Advanced Fertility Services, for their individual contributions to the care of the many couples who have sought our assistance in their quest to have a baby. - H.D.M.

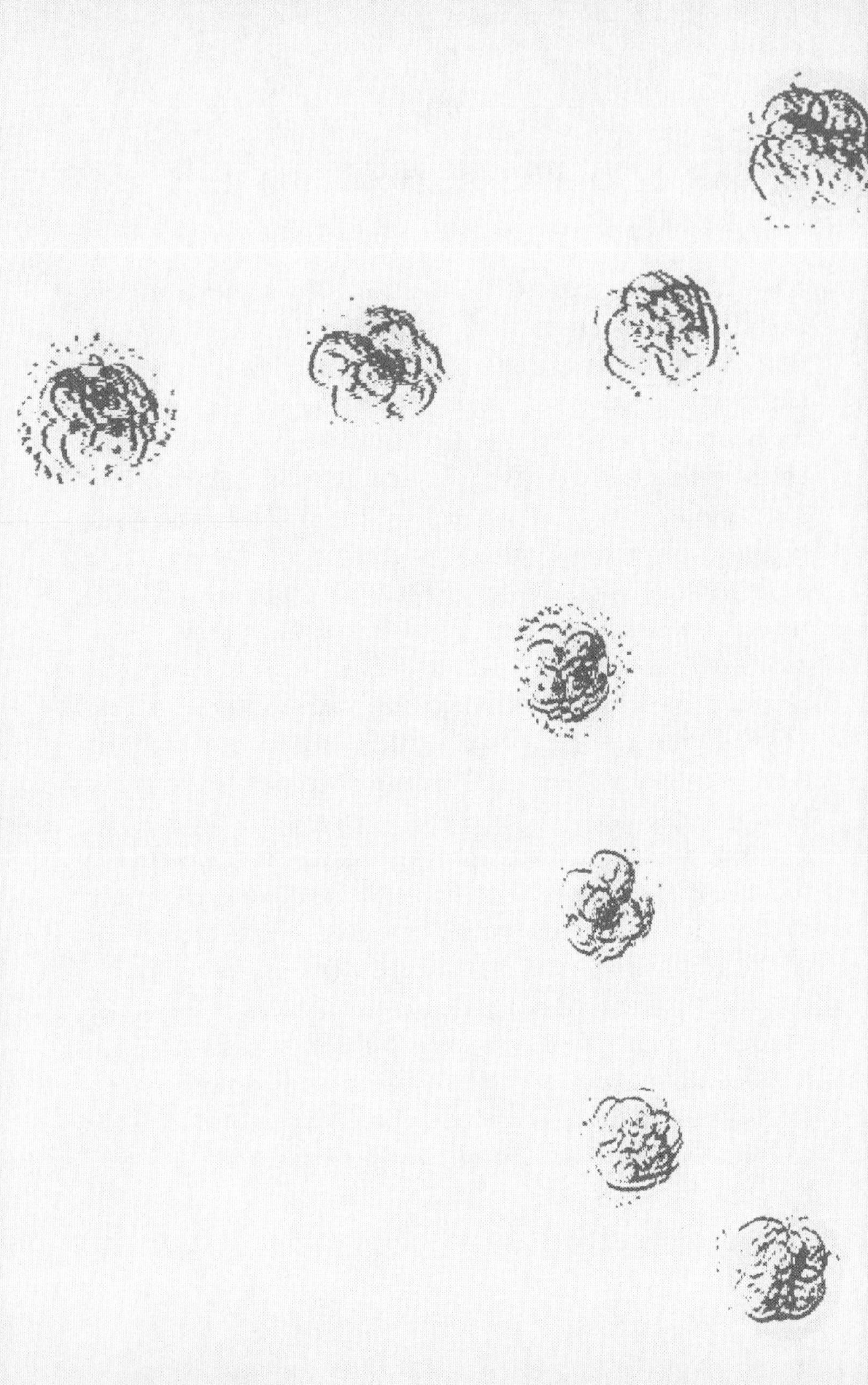

TABLE OF CONTENTS

INTRODUCTION

"What I see in Nature is a magnificent structure that we can comprehend only very imperfectly, and that must fill a thinking person with a feeling of humility."

~Albert Einstein

If you are reading this book, chances are that you have traveled a difficult road in your quest to have a baby. You are probably disappointed, frustrated and afraid that you may never succeed in conceiving the child that you want so dearly. Month after month, your pregnancy tests keep turning out negative and you don't understand why. Frustration and anger may cause you to blame yourself or your partner for your failure to become pregnant.

What makes the situation even more difficult is that you may not know where to turn. First, you face the difficult and confusing task of selecting a doctor or a fertility clinic in the hopes of finding the cause of the "problem," as well as finding a miraculous cure that will promptly result in a pregnancy. Once that choice has been made, you may wonder which diagnostic tests to undergo. You are fearful that the results of these tests may indicate that you will never be able to conceive. As soon as your diagnostic tests are completed, you are pressured to make an educated decision about which fertility treatment you should pursue. However, you feel insecure about making a choice, as you lack the necessary information. You might even be asking yourself whether you are "desperate" enough to resort to the high-tech fertility treatments that may be needed to become pregnant.

The worst part of it is that you have come to realize that the process of trying to have a baby is beyond your control. This realization is both frightening and depressing. Your inability to become pregnant dominates all your waking thoughts, and cloaks your otherwise happy life in despair. It is critical to recognize that 15-25% of couples are, like yourself, unable to have a baby. They share the same concerns, anxieties and fears. They suffer, much as you do, being an unwilling passenger on the same monthly emotional roller coaster. Although you suffer privately, you are not alone.

When I wrote the first edition of The Pregnancy Prescription more than ten years ago, one of my goals was to ensure that infertile couples understood that their inability to conceive was not a medical condition that required the traditional diagnostic approach used by physicians to formulate treatment for a disease. In most cases, the actual causes of infertility cannot be determined by traditional diagnostic tests, as most of these factors occur on the cellular and molecular levels. Therefore, I advocated the "success-oriented" approach for infertile couples. The "success-oriented" approach begins with a couple first undergoing a limited number of basic noninvasive tests to rule out major "roadblocks" to conception. If no major problems are found, a progressive course of treatment is initiated that would augment and amplify the natural process of conception. I also suggested that *In Vitro* Fertilization (IVF) be used earlier in the process, both diagnostically and therapeutically, so that cellular events such as fertilization problems and abnormalities of embryo growth could be studied and treated. Furthermore, IVF bypasses all the internal steps necessary for joining the egg and sperm at the molecular level, at which any number of otherwise undetectable problems may prevent successful conception. I am happy to report that in the past ten years, most fertility specialists have abandoned the traditional diagnostic orientation and have embraced the success-oriented model of infertility treatment.

In the past ten years, one of the most significant advances in reproductive medicine has been in the area of genetic analysis of living embryos. This has given us an unprecedented understanding of why conception fails so often, despite the existence of ideal conditions. It is crucial that couples struggling with infertility understand that the genetic content of an embryo ultimately controls whether or not it will become a healthy baby. More simply stated, conception is a natural phenomenon that cannot be influenced in any way by a person's lifestyle, diet or general state of health. As long as eggs and sperm are present, pregnancy is possible if the genetic content of the embryo is perfectly configured so as to produce a healthy baby. If there is a single genetic defect, 99% of the time the embryo will cease to grow. This is the process of natural selection, which is Nature's way of ensuring the birth of healthy babies. If couples recognize that Nature ultimately controls if and when a pregnancy occurs, they will be able to persevere with treatment. It is critical that these couples not feel frustrated or harbor feelings of guilt as in many cases, even with the most ideal fertility treatment, achieving a pregnancy can take time.

I sincerely hope that after reading this book couples will have a new perspective on infertility. The reality is that the process of conception is so complex that it is far beyond human comprehension and control. After 30 years of treating infertile couples, I have come to recognize that the more I learn about the process of conception, the more miraculous and mysterious it becomes. There are no "absolute truths" in the diagnosis and treatment of infertile couples. Couples with a poor prognosis for becoming pregnant often conceive, whereas others, who should be able to become pregnant easily, do not. I have come to believe that conception is ultimately governed by Nature. I hope that after reading The Pregnancy Prescription, infertile couples will gain an understanding of the underlying mechanisms by which Nature controls conception. Perhaps then they will come to share my belief that infertility is the failure of a natural process, rather than a disease. As a result of this new insight, they will not feel, in any way, diminished or defective by their inability to conceive. Rather, it is my hope that this newfound knowledge will provide couples with the necessary resilience to persevere with treatment until a satisfactory outcome is attained.

Hugh D. Melnick, M.D., F.A.C.O.G

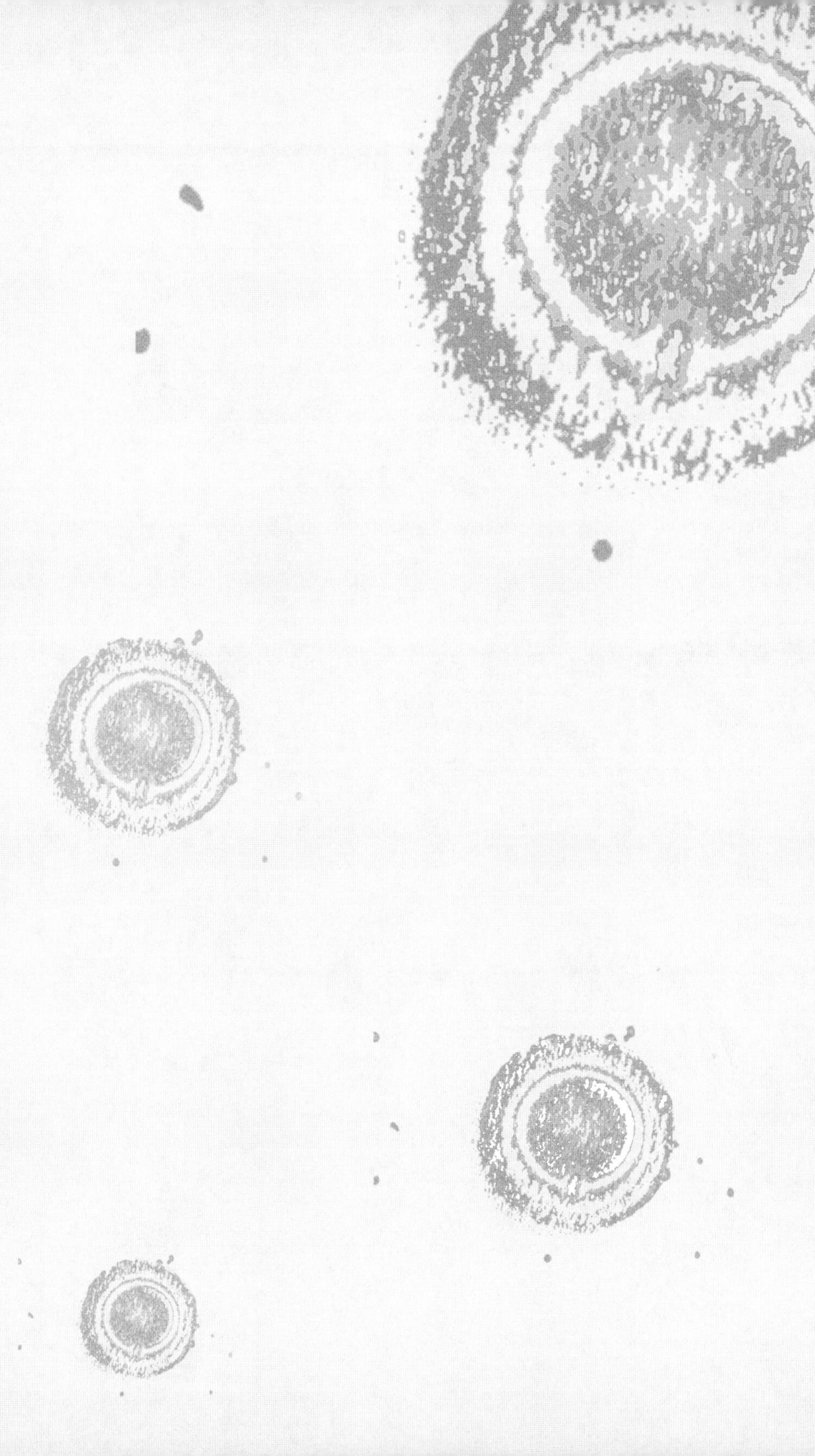

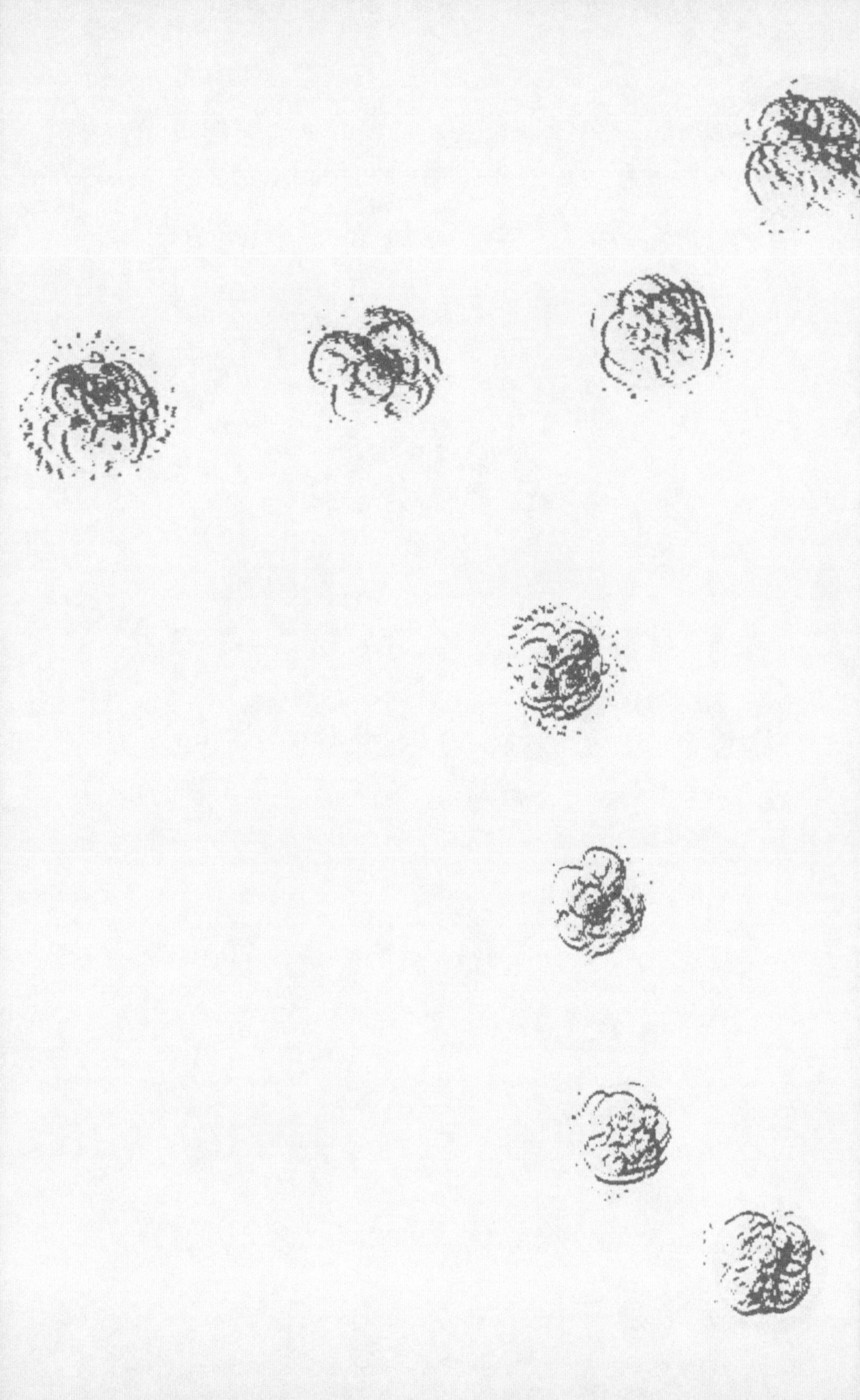

CHAPTER 1

NATURAL REPRODUCTION:

How The Process Should Work

If you are trying to have a baby, chances are good that you already understand the basics of reproduction. What you may not realize, however, is that conception is like a game of dominoes: if all the pieces are in perfect alignment, each will fall in its proper sequence until none is left standing and conception occurs. But if even one single piece is slightly out of line, the whole process will fail.

This quick review of oocyte (egg) development, fertilization and implantation may help you better understand some of the factors that might be working against your attempts to conceive.

OOCYTE DEVELOPMENT

A woman's menstrual cycle is the result of an elegant system of hormonal signals that is self-programmed to produce a mature, chromosomally and genetically appropriate egg during each cycle.

A LIFETIME SUPPLY

A baby girl is born with all the eggs she will ever have in her lifetime. These eggs, which usually number about 500,000, develop while the fetus is still in the mother's uterus, and then remain in a resting state in the ovaries until the girl reaches puberty at 11 to 14 years of age. Once she begins menstruating, about 1,000 of her eggs will become stimulated each month. Of these, only one (or rarely, two) will become mature and be released from the ovary each month. The remainder regress and die. On average, a woman's lifetime supply of eggs will be diminished by about 12,000 per year. Over a 30-year period, she may lose as many as 360,000 of the original 500,000.

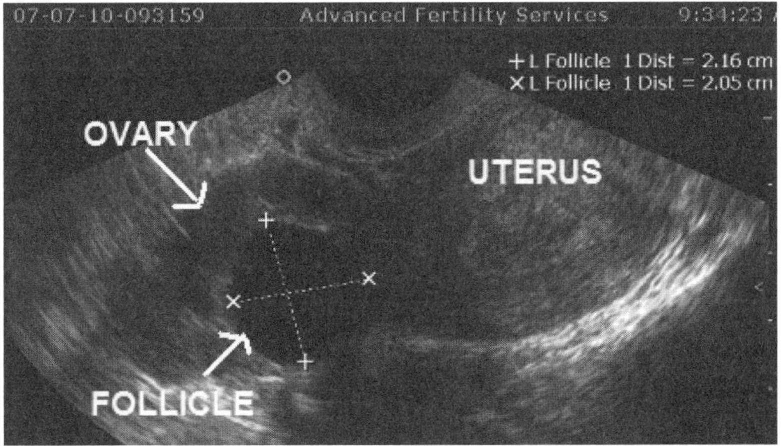

Fig. 1. ***A sonogram showing the ovary with a mature follicle, with a diameter of 20 mm, containing an egg inside.***

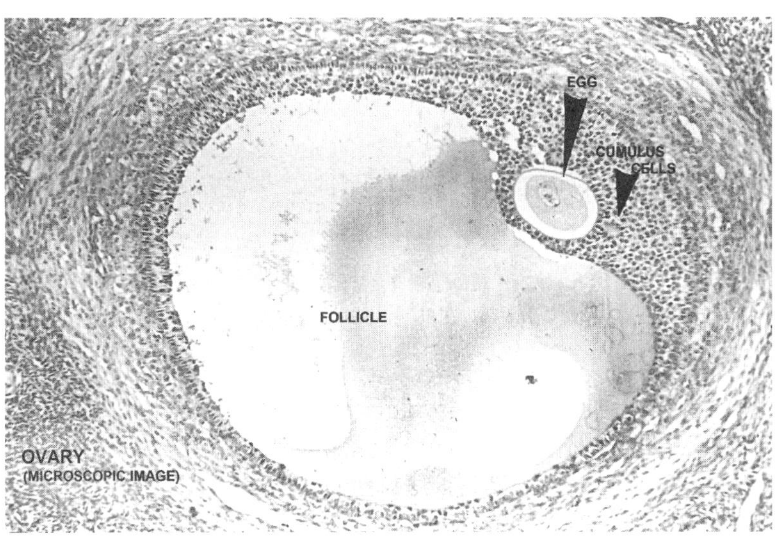

Fig. 2. ***Microscopic view of*** Fig. 1, ***showing an ovarian follicle containing a mature egg prior to its release at time of ovulation.***

THE INITIAL STAGE OF EGG DEVELOPMENT

The key hormones responsible for egg development are Follicle-Stimulating Hormone (FSH) and Luteinizing Hormone (LH). Both FSH and LH are produced by the pituitary gland, a tiny almond-shaped gland located at the base of the brain. The pituitary gland is controlled, in turn, by the hypothalamus—an area in the brain that is situated directly above the pituitary gland. Under normal circumstances, the hypothalamus sends monthly signals to the pituitary gland to produce FSH and LH, so that ovulation occurs each month.

The first half of a woman's monthly ovulatory cycle consists of roughly a two-week period of egg development, during which FSH and LH cause the egg gradually to mature into a state that is capable of being fertilized by a sperm. The entire cycle is ultimately governed by the hormone estrogen, which is produced by cells in the ovary called granulosa cells, which surround each egg. At the beginning of the cycle of ovulation, a woman's estrogen level is low, so the pituitary gland releases high levels of FSH. As FSH stimulates egg growth, the estrogen-producing granulosa cells surrounding it proliferate, increasing a woman's estrogen levels in parallel with the development of the egg. As increasing levels of estrogen turn off FSH production, the body self-regulates the initial stages of egg development, so that it "knows" when the egg has completed its initial stage of maturation.

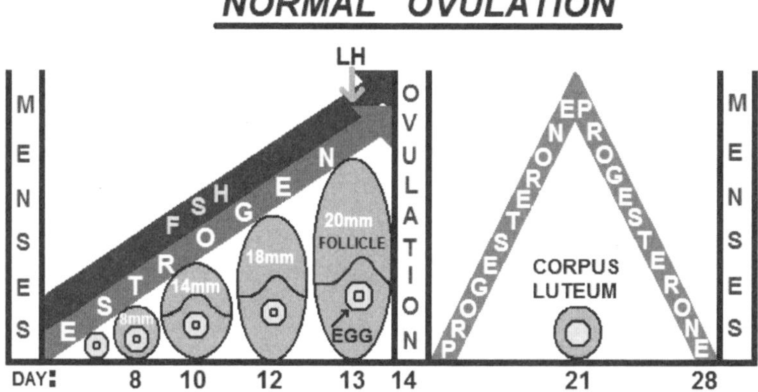

Fig. 3. *Follicle Development*

Once an ovarian follicle starts to be stimulated, it becomes the "dominant follicle" and begins growing by about 2 millimeters (mm) per day. The egg is considered to be in the fertile zone when the follicle measures 20 mm, which is slightly less than 1 inch. Although the mature egg itself is microscopic (approximately 100 mature eggs will fit on the head of a pin), the growth of the follicle—the ovarian sac in which the egg grows—can be tracked through ultrasound.

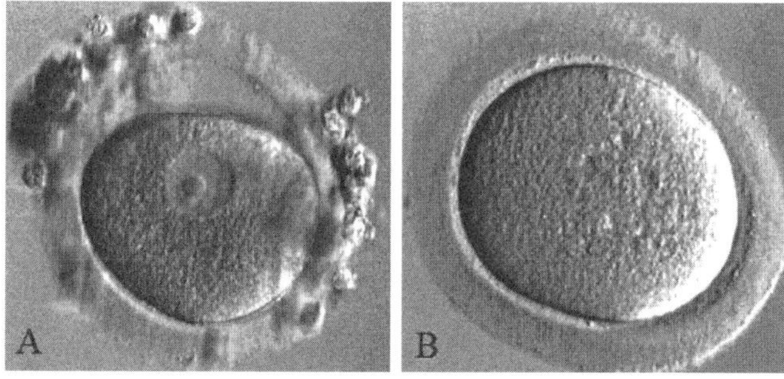

Fig.4 A. Egg at the Germinal Vessicle Stage (most immature). B. Egg at the MI stage, 24-36 hours prior to full maturation. Both eggs still have 46 chromosomes and have not yet undergone reduction division to the mature egg status of 23 chromosomes.

THE FINAL STEPS TO EGG MATURITY

When a woman's estrogen level reaches a critically high point, it not only causes the termination of the initial stage of egg development, it simultaneously provides a signal to the hypothalamus that the egg is mature and is ready to undergo the final process that enables it to be fertilized. The high levels of estrogen then trigger a different center in the hypothalamus to stimulate the pituitary gland to release vast stores of LH, which causes the final step of egg maturation to occur. This outpouring of LH is called the LH surge.

The urine home ovulation kits that so many women use detect this LH surge, which actually indicates the start of the period of optimum fertility. This final stage, a process called reduction division (meiosis), is critical for normal fertilization to occur. The process of reduction division reduces the number of chromosomes contained in the egg from 46 (humans normally have 46 chromosomes per cell, arranged in 23 identical pairs) to 23 single chromosomes. Since there are 23 chromosomes in a mature, normal sperm cell, when sperm and egg are united through fertilization the resulting embryo should acquire its full normal complement of 46 chromosomes: 23 from the biological mother via the egg and 23 from the sperm of the biological father.

More frequently than not, too much or too little genetic material may end up in the embryo. There are multiple reasons for an embryo with an abnormal number of chromosomes: the problem can result from an abnormal egg, an abnormal sperm, or an abnormality in the process of fertilization itself. Since the process of egg development and fertilization is so complex, it is no wonder that the vast majority of embryos are genetically abnormal! ***The most important fact to remember is that such genetic errors are, by far, the most common causes of non-conception and miscarriages.***

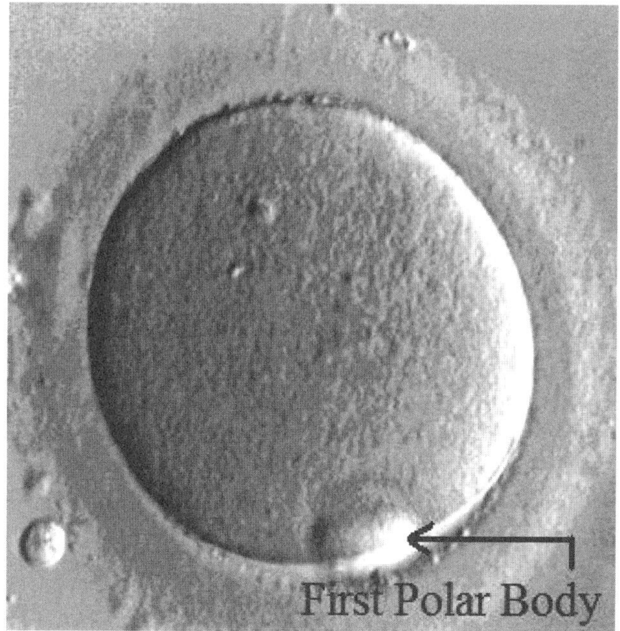

Fig. 5. ***A mature oocyte at the MII stage. Maturity is indicated by the presence of a "polar body"—the round structure found at the edge of the egg in the 5 o'clock position. This polar body contains the 23 chromosomes that have been discarded as a result of reduction division. This is the end point of egg maturity.***

OOCYTE RELEASE

About 36 hours after the LH surge, the follicle in which the egg is contained will burst. The egg is released, along with its surrounding granulosa cells and the follicular fluid, which contains a variety of proteins and hormones.

It is remarkable that the final step of egg maturation (meiosis) and the ultimate release of the mature egg are both governed by the same hormone, LH. I am in awe of the manner in which Nature ensures that an egg is released only when it is ready to be fertilized. Although the development of the mature egg on its path to fertilization results from a beautifully synchronized ebb and flow of hormones from two distant organs—the brain and the ovaries—Nature cannot guarantee that the genetic constitution of an egg, sperm or embryo will be sufficiently perfect to create a healthy baby. In fact, the vast number of embryos created, either naturally or in the IVF lab, are genetically imperfect. This high incidence of embryonic genetic abnormalities explains why conception, either natural or through fertility treatment, is far from 100% successful, even under the most perfect of conditions.

FERTILIZATION: SURVIVAL OF THE FITTEST

The high levels of estrogen that help to signal the LH surge and bring about the release of the egg also serve to increase the quality and quantity of mucus in the woman's cervix, uterus and Fallopian tubes. The mucus acts as a preservative for the sperm that are ejaculated into the vagina and are strong enough to reach the opening of the womb.

When a man ejaculates, only 10% of his sperm actually reaches the cervical mucus. The remainder of the sperm perish in the vagina, which, due to its acidity, is not well suited to supporting their longevity. From that point on, "survival of the fittest" is the rule: the farther up through the genital tract the sperm travel, the fewer survive. In fact, some studies have shown that even if as many as 100-200 million sperm have been ejaculated into a woman's vagina, only 500 live sperm may arrive in each of her Fallopian tubes. Those that do reach their ultimate destination are not only the strongest, but also the fastest: studies have shown that sperm may arrive at the outer ends of the Fallopian tubes as soon as 10 minutes after insemination.

EARLY IS BETTER THAN LATE

Since sperm have been proven capable of surviving as long as five to seven days in the mucus-lined genital tract or uterine cavity, the precise timing of intercourse is not critical for fertilization. This knowledge should help reduce the psychological pressure for couples that mistakenly believe it is necessary to achieve split-second accuracy in the timing of intercourse for pregnancy to occur. Recent studies indicate that pregnancy is most likely to occur when intercourse takes place in the period just before the egg has been released. Cervical mucus can start to become hostile to sperm beginning about 18 hours after the egg has been released (or 54-58 hours after the LH surge), and once that has occurred, the sperm can no longer survive.

WHERE EGG MEETS SPERM

In certain species, the female anatomy seems designed to help increase the chances for fertilization and conception. In female rabbits, for example, the Fallopian tube surrounds the ovary. When a rabbit releases her eggs they are deposited directly into her Fallopian tube, where fertilization takes place. This anatomical advantage is a likely explanation for why rabbits are so fertile and is the reason that the phrase "multiply like rabbits" was coined.

The human female anatomy is quite different from that of a female rabbit. The tiny (less than 1 mm) opening of a human Fallopian tube lies at least 4 to 6 centimeters (1.5-2.5 inches) away from the ovary. ***It is anatomically impossible for a human egg to be caught by the Fallopian tube as it is released from the ovary.***

So how does it get there? The most likely explanation is that after the follicle ruptures, the egg and follicular fluid accumulate in a pool in the area behind the uterus known as the Pouch of Douglas (or cul de sac). Since sperm that successfully travel to the ends of the Fallopian tubes are also found in the Pouch of Douglas, we believe that this may be where the egg and sperm unite. The Fallopian tubes have sticky, finger-like projections at the ends called fimbria that dip into this pool of fluid in the cul de sac. The egg/cumulus cell complex adhere to this surface and are drawn into the Fallopian tube.

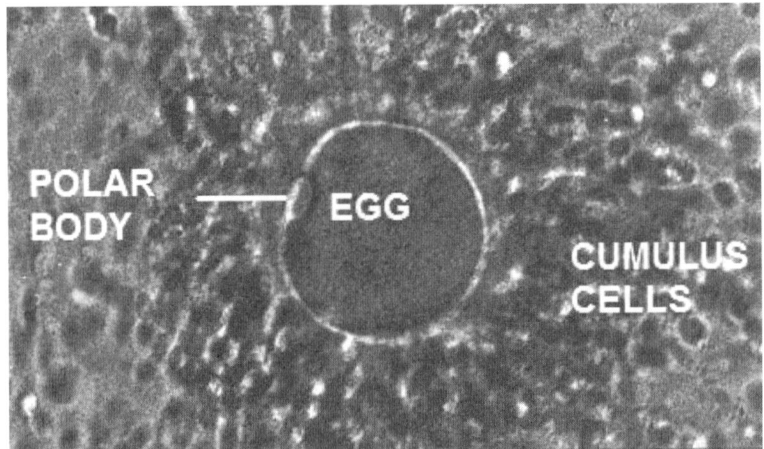

Fig. 6. ***The egg as it appears to the embryologist when it is first removed from the ovarian follicle.***

When eggs are released from the ovary, I believe that an attachment takes place between the fimbria and the cumulus cells, and that the fimbria actually suck the egg/cumulus structure out of the cul de sac and into the opening of the tube either through very fine muscular contractions or via propulsion by the cilia (hair-like cells) that line the Fallopian tubes.

At Advanced Fertility Services in New York City, we developed a procedure called Intraperitoneal Insemination (IPI) many years ago. In IPI, we injected small numbers of sperm through the wall of the vagina and into the cul de sac fluid soon after ovulation had taken place. This technique, which was utilized in the late 1980s, resulted in pregnancies for a number of women who were unable to conceive via normal intrauterine insemination. This may be because the sperm were placed directly into the area where the eggs had been deposited, making it easier for them to come into direct contact with the egg. Or, the process may protect the sperm from anti-sperm antibodies or other toxic substances that may be secreted by the uterus or circulated through the Fallopian tubes. Intraperitoneal Insemination is described in greater detail in Chapter 6. This technique has not been commonly used since the development of a technique called Intracytoplasmic Sperm Injection (ICSI), which is a more direct method of fertilizing eggs when only small numbers of sperm are available. This procedure is discussed in the chapters on male infertility and the IVF laboratory (Chapters 9 and 10).

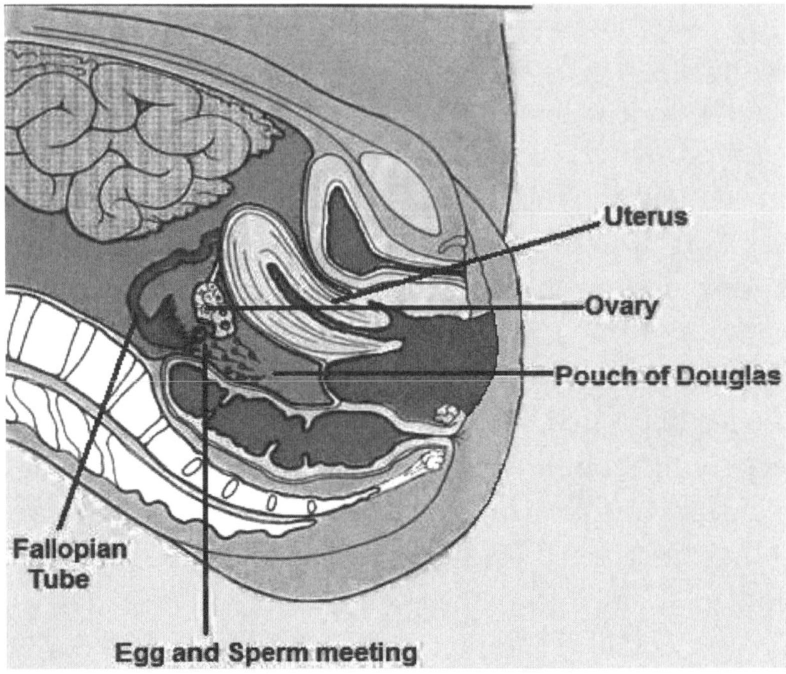

Fig. 7. ***Diagram of the process of fertilization that occurs in the female reproductive system.***

BECOMING AN EMBRYO

When sperm and egg meet during the initial stages of fertilization, hundreds of sperm may attempt to penetrate the thick layers of granulosa cells that surround the egg. Those sperm that swim with a sufficiently strong velocity will latch onto receptors on the surface of the egg, similar to the way a spaceship latches onto a landing site on a space station. After a sperm has locked on, a reaction begins that causes it to release a package of enzymes (the acrosome) located in the head of the sperm to help it penetrate the outer shell of the egg, which is known as the zona pellucida.

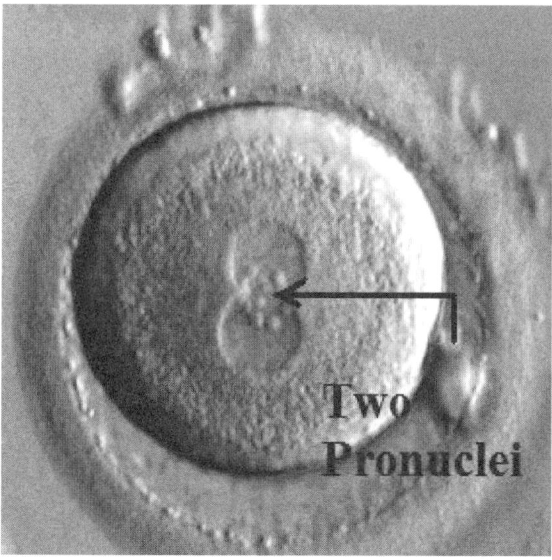

Fig. 8. ***The earliest embryo, 18 hours after fertilization. Two pronuclei are present in the center, indicating that the genetic material of the egg and sperm have joined together.***

Once the first sperm has successfully penetrated the shell, all other sperm will be blocked from gaining entry. If an egg were to become fertilized by more than one sperm (polyspermia), the resulting embryo would contain more than the normal amount of genetic material, making it incapable of surviving. Embryos created as a result of polyspermy always miscarry at a very early stage of development.

If there has been successful fertilization, two pronuclei (round, circular structures) will be visible inside the egg, about 18 hours later. One of these circular structures contains genetic material from the egg (23 chromosomes), and the other holds the same amount of genetic material from the sperm. The two pronuclei then break down and fuse, providing the embryo with its full complement of 46 chromosomes.

Once the pronuclei have broken down, the embryo begins to divide. Approximately 48 hours after fertilization the embryo will consist of two to four cells; by 72 hours post-fertilization, there will be six to eight cells. At that point, cell division begins to occur rapidly. Four to five days after fertilization, the embryo will consist of more than 1000 cells within the zona pellucida. This is called the morula stage.

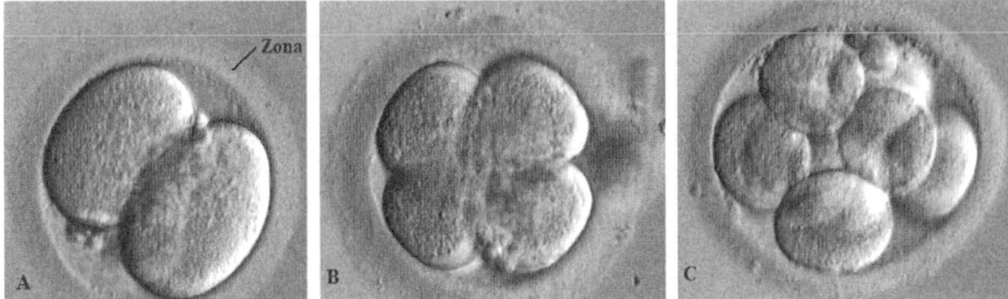

Fig. 9. A. ***Two-cell embryo (24 hours).***
B. ***Four-cell embryo (48 hours).***
C. ***Eight-cell embryo (72 hours).***

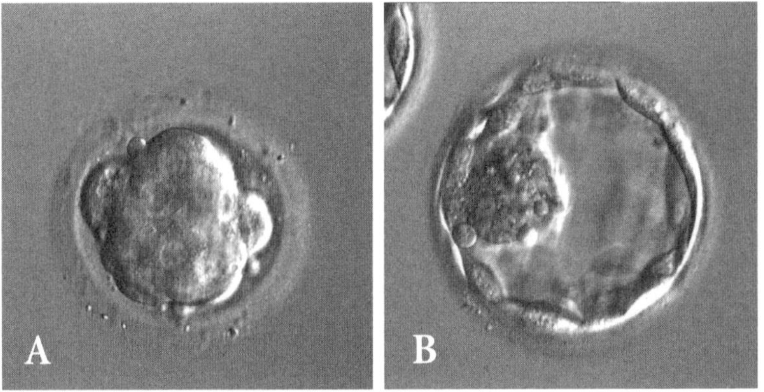

Fig. 10. A. ***Morula stage embryo, four days after fertilization.***
B. Blastocyst stage embryo, five days after fertilization.

IMPLANTATION

As cell division occurs, the embryo makes its way from the fimbria through the length of the Fallopian tube and into the uterus. By the time it has reached its destination, the embryo is in the blastocyst stage, at which time the zona pellucida breaks down and the embryo "hatches," or bursts out of its shell. Hatching is critical, because the shell limits the ability of the embryo to expand and prevents it from implanting into the lining of the uterus. Implantation usually occurs five to seven days after fertilization.

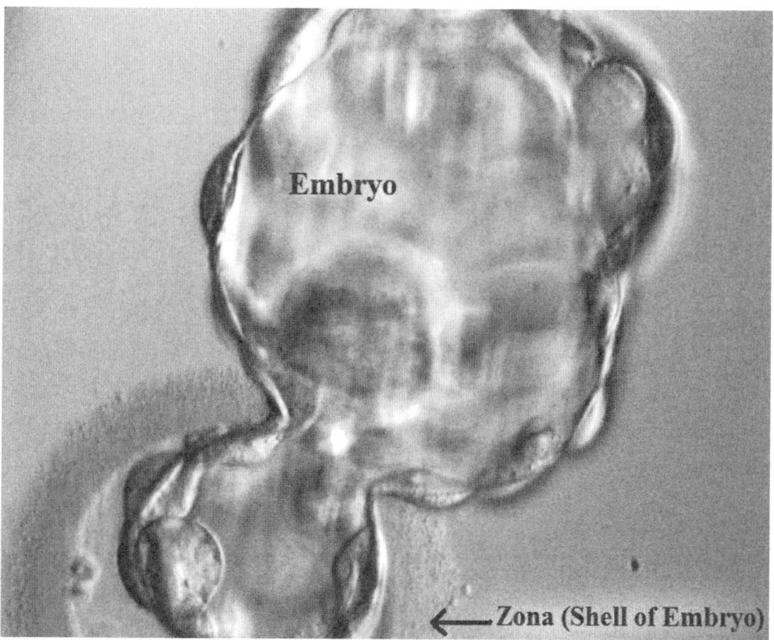

Fig. 11. ***The embryo hatching out of its shell prior to implantation in the uterus. Just think of a chick hatching out of its eggshell, and you will visualize this process.***

SUMMARY

The human reproductive system is set up in a very logical, nearly foolproof manner, so that we should be equipped to reproduce quite efficiently. Unfortunately, even when all factors fall into line perfectly and the sperm and egg join together, a single, minor glitch at the genetic level of the process, more often than not, prevents the ultimate objective— a normal, healthy ongoing pregnancy. In Chapter 2, you will learn more about these glitches and how they may be sabotaging you in your struggle to conceive.

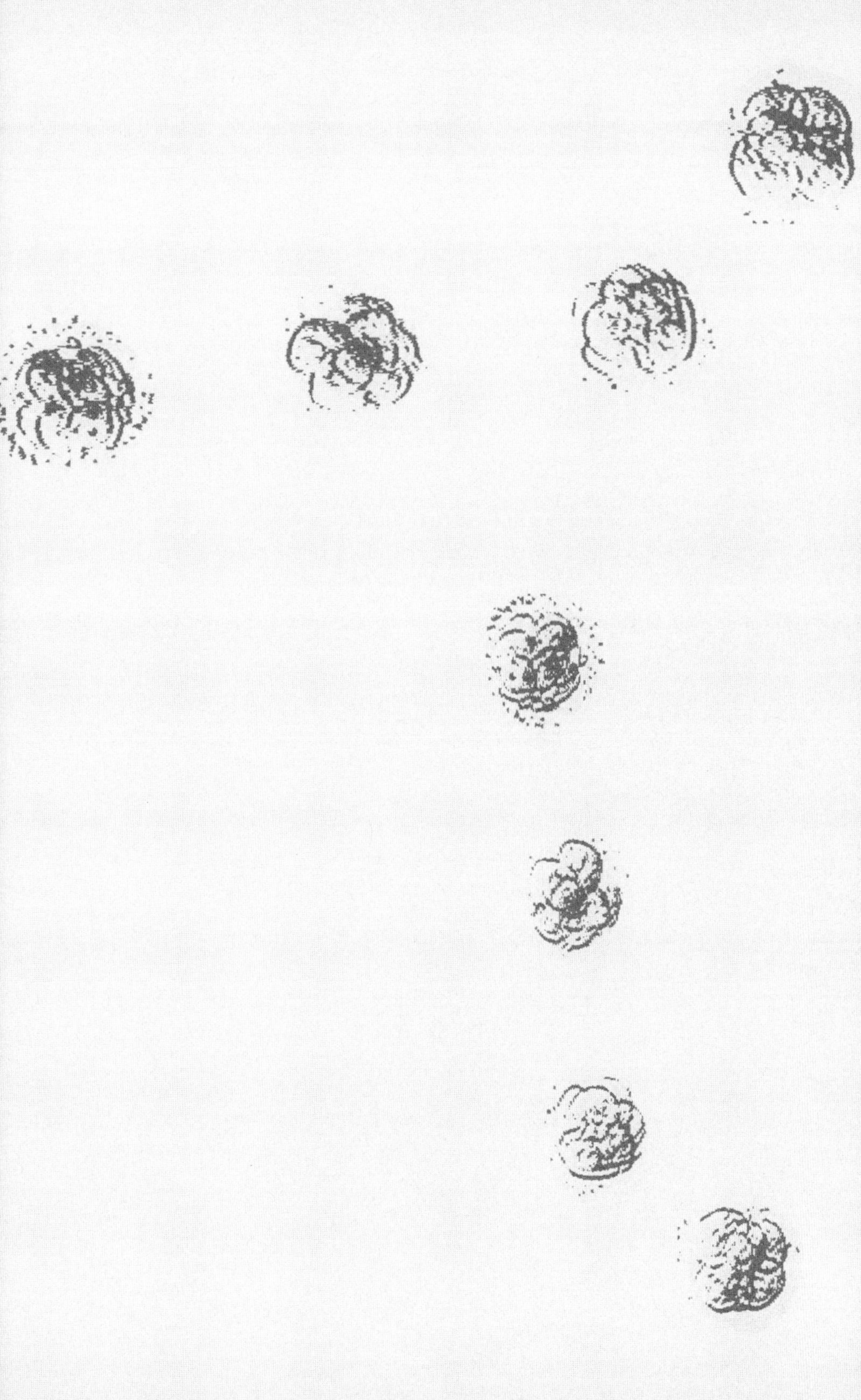

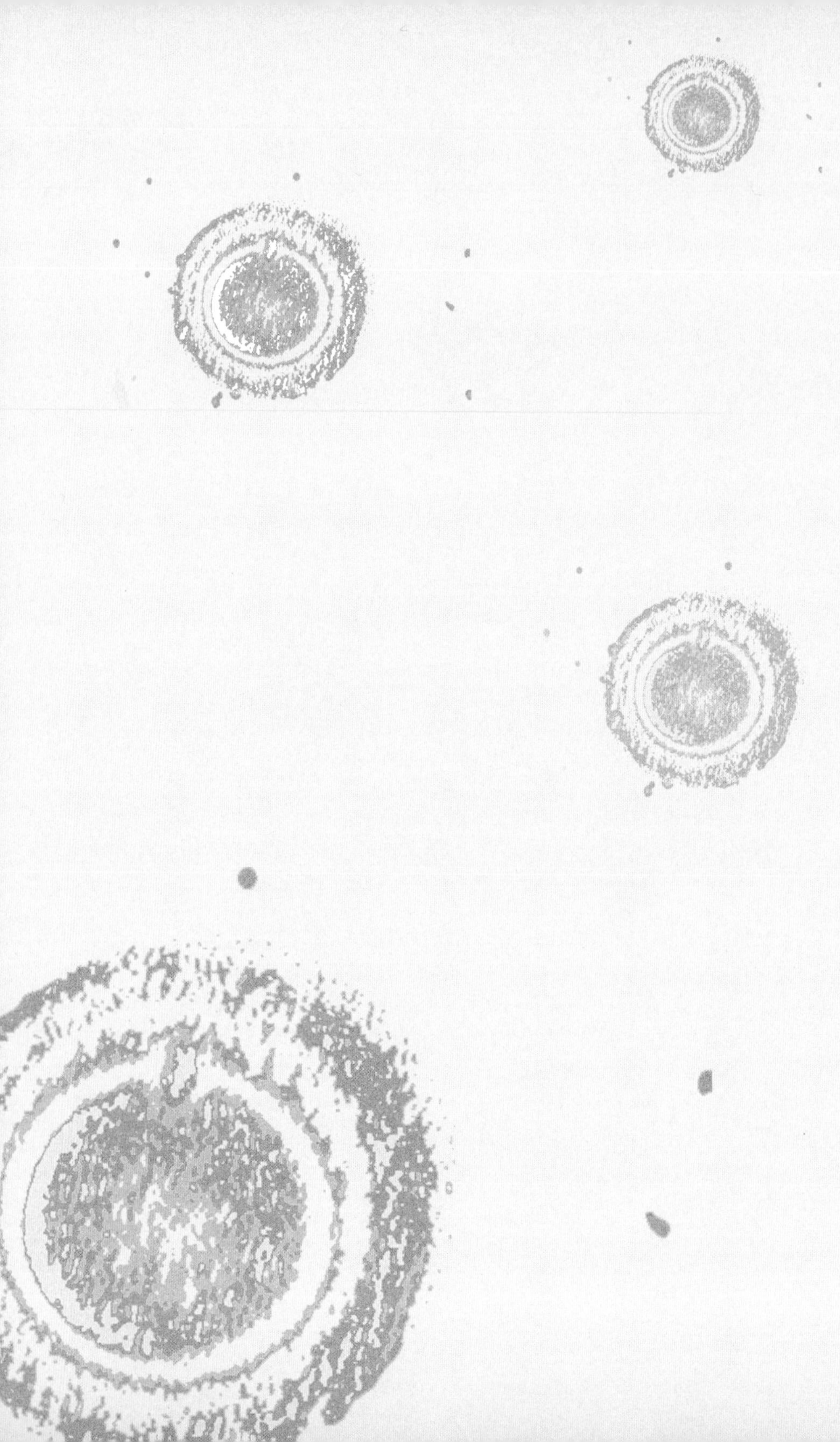

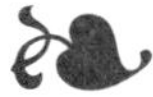

CHAPTER 2

BARRIERS TO CONCEPTION: *What Might Be Going Wrong*

The first thing that you and your partner must understand is that your inability to conceive is not a result of anything that you have or have not done. A faulty diet, overly vigorous exercise or high levels of stress—though not ideal for your overall health—are not barriers to conception. **Apart from having sex during a woman's 72-hour window of fertility, conception is beyond human control. The reason for this is that the vast majority of embryos fail to implant because of abnormalities that are present in their chromosomal or genetic content.** These genetic abnormalities occur when the complex process of fertilization goes awry. It may be surprising to learn that, far more often than not, the fertilization process does not work properly, resulting in a genetically flawed embryo—which cannot possibly develop into a perfectly formed, healthy baby. Therefore the failure of a genetically compromised embryo to implant is a blessing in disguise. The ability of Nature to allow only the most genetically perfect embryos to survive is the quintessential safeguard that ensures the birth of healthy babies. Therefore you must rid yourself of any thoughts of guilt for your inability to conceive. It is ironic that factors that can be controlled, such as good nutrition or the maintenance of a healthy lifestyle, do not enhance fertility. Taking prenatal vitamins, limiting caffeine intake or abstaining from alcoholic beverages will **not** make a woman more fertile, no more than avoiding hot baths and wearing boxer shorts will increase a man's sperm count. The truth is that most of the information that is published in the popular press about the effects of diet and lifestyle on fertility and miscarriage are more fiction than scientific fact.

THE ODDS

Since each cell in our bodies contains 23 pairs of chromosomes and each chromosome carries between 500 and 3,000 individual genes, the potential for a genetic abnormality in a newly created embryo is huge. Fortunately, Nature doesn't allow the vast majority of embryos with chromosomal or genetic abnormalities to survive to the point that would make a woman's period late or even result in a positive pregnancy test. Instead, these embryos self-destruct as a result of natural selection, which is Nature's fail-safe mechanism that prevents the birth of abnormal babies.

It is important to realize that the vast majority of every woman's eggs, as well as a man's sperm, can develop abnormal numbers of chromosomes (aneuploidy) or genetic mutations. It is impossible to test for these mutations because of the tremendous number of genes present: each of the 23 chromosomes in a mature egg (or sperm) has large numbers of gene sites on it, each with a unique molecular DNA structure. Should the DNA structure of any gene be altered, a lethal mutation can be produced. This would cause the embryo to fail to develop past the point of implantation. For this reason, even if all of the steps leading to fertilization and implantation take place perfectly, *any* embryo has only a 20% chance of developing into a clinically observable pregnancy.

Although Nature causes about 80% of potential embryos to "miscarry" before a pregnancy becomes evident, the 20% that remain cannot all be considered to be genetically sound. An additional 25-35% may last long enough to cause a positive pregnancy test, but will prove incapable of surviving for more than a few days. A pregnancy that ends at a very early point in time—by one week after an initial positive pregnancy test—is called a "biochemical pregnancy." Pregnancies that survive for six to eight weeks after the last menstrual period are termed "clinical miscarriages." A gestational sac may be seen within the uterus, but the fetus does not develop. This very common type of clinical miscarriage is called a "blighted ovum." These miscarriages are caused exclusively by genetic abnormalities that originated at the time of fertilization.

Once a fetal heartbeat can be detected on an ultrasound examination, usually at the time that a woman's period is two weeks late, the prospective parents can begin to breathe easier. At that point, the chance of miscarriage declines from 35% to 5%.

NORMAL HUMAN CHROMOSOMES

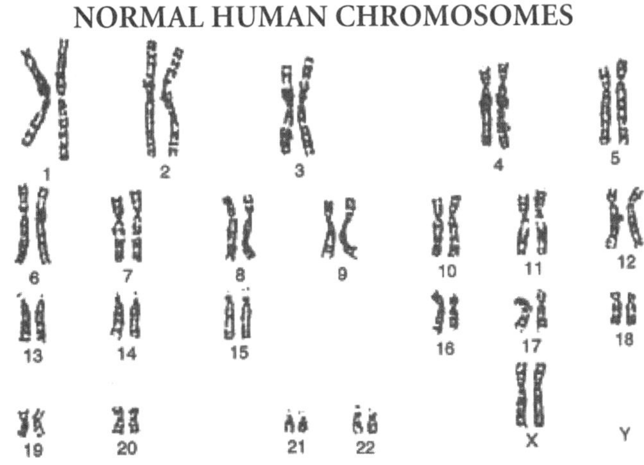

Fig. 1. ***The chromosomal content of a normal female. There are 2 X chromosomes (and no Y chromosomes) indicating that the embryo is a female. There are also 22 other exactly matched pairs of chromosomes. Note that the lines on each chromosome are in perfect alignment. These lines indicate individual gene sites.***

HUMAN CHROMOSOMES AND GENE SITES

Chromosome Number	Number of Genes on the Chromosome
1	3,148
2	902
3	1,436
4	453
5	609
6	1,585
7	1,824
8	781
9	1,229
10	1,312
11	405
12	1,330
13	623
14	886
15	676
16	898
17	1,367
18	365
19	1,553
20	816
21	446
22	595
X (sex chromosome)	1,093
Y (sex chromosome)	125

Fig. 2. ***The number of individual gene sites on each human chromosome. There are approximately 24,457 known genes.***

WHAT'S AGE GOT TO DO WITH IT?

Even prior to birth, a woman's lifetime supply of eggs lies dormant in her ovaries. Her eggs, which contain her genetic material—the DNA found in the chromosomes—remain in a resting state until puberty begins, at which time ovulation starts. A woman is most fertile during her teenage years. This is because the structure of her DNA molecules that comprise the individual genes on each chromosome is held firmly in place by electrochemical bonds. These bonds are the "glue" that holds the DNA strands together in their proper alignment. As a woman ages, the electrochemical bonds naturally weaken and become less able to maintain the structure of individual genes in the exact shape and configuration necessary for the creation of a genetically perfect offspring. These alterations, known as genetic mutations, are probably among the major factors responsible for the reduction in fertility experienced by women as they grow older.

In contrast to a woman being born with a lifetime supply of eggs, men are born with cells that produce fresh sperm on a continuous basis after the onset of puberty. These cells produce new spermatozoa in 72-96 days. This means that the DNA contained within any individual sperm can be no more than two-to-three months old at any time, and the electrochemical bonds that hold sperm DNA in position are less likely to deteriorate.

MORE GENETIC MAYHEM

An embryo frequently ends up with either more or less than the normal number of 46 chromosomes, which are arranged in each cell of the human body as 23 matching pairs. When an embryo contains an abnormal number of chromosomal strands, it is almost always so flawed that it is impossible for it to develop into a normal baby. This condition is called "aneuploidy." Along with genetic mutations, aneuploidy is the other major cause of the failure of an embryo to implant. Fortunately, Nature has the ability to detect when an embryo has genetic abnormalities, and in that situation, the unhealthy embryo's continued growth and development are inevitably terminated. This remarkable process of natural selection ensures that 99% of babies are perfectly formed.

Aneuploidy can be created both at the time of reduction division of the egg (meiosis) and at the time of fertilization. During meiosis, the egg can be left with too few or too many chromosomal strands. Consequently, at the time of fertilization, an aneuploidic embryo is inevitably formed. The other way that a genetically abnormal embryo can be formed is when a mature egg, with a normal chromosomal number, is fertilized by a sperm. Although the embryo seems to be off to a good start, the problem occurs a bit later in the process of fertilization, when chromosomes belonging to both the egg and the sperm are paired up prior to its first division. The embryo is then left with too many or too few chromosomes. In most cases, having too many or too few chromosomes is "lethal" for an embryo. The end result is that the embryo will fail to implant in the uterus, or a biochemical pregnancy or clinical miscarriage will occur. Embryos can be tested for aneuploidy when they are produced in the IVF laboratory using a technique called Preimplantation Genetic Diagnosis (PGD). Embryonic genetic testing will be discussed in Chapter 12.

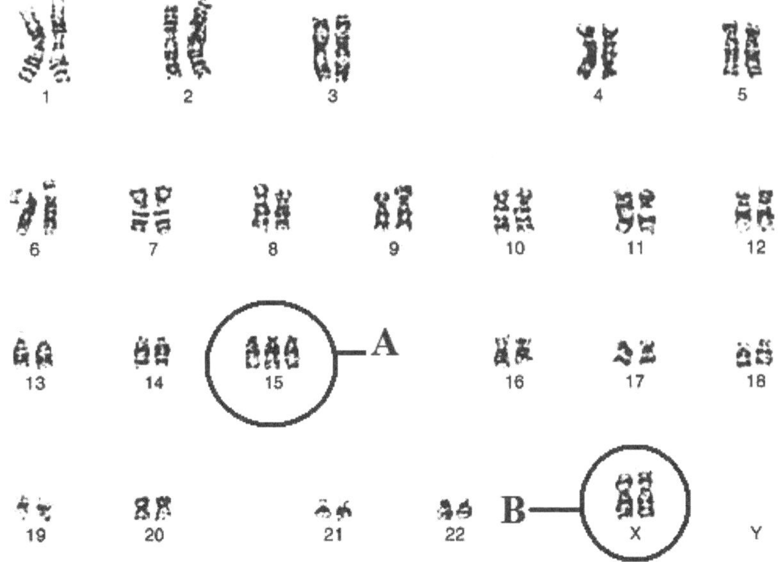

Fig. 3. ***Genetic analysis of a cell from a miscarriage. (A) indicates an extra chromosome #15, which is not compatible with life. (B) indicates the female sex of the embryo.***

AS IF THAT WEREN'T ENOUGH …

In addition to genetic abnormalities, there are many other factors that can prevent conception:

For The Woman

- Hormonal imbalances may prevent the woman from producing a viable egg.
- The uterine lining may not develop sufficiently to be capable of sustaining a pregnancy.
- The woman may have fibroids or another uterine abnormality that interferes with uterine blood supply and prevents the embryo from implanting.
- The woman's cervical mucus may be hostile to her partner's sperm (either due to infection or an antibody reaction).
- The woman's eggs may not be able to be fertilized. This

may occur if the zona pellucida is too thick or if sperm cannot penetrate it.

- The woman's Fallopian tubes may be blocked, preventing access to the eggs by the sperm.
- The Fallopian tubes may not function properly in picking up or transporting the eggs.

For The Man

- Too few sperm may be produced.
- The motility (movement) of the sperm may be insufficient to move the sperm from the vagina to the cervix, or beyond that to the Fallopian tubes.
- The sperm may not be able to bind onto an egg.
- The sperm may not have the enzymes (acrosome) to "eat" their way into the egg.
- The sperm may not have the velocity (speed or energy) to penetrate cumulus cells surrounding the egg.
- The sperm may contain abnormal genetic material.

SUMMARY

After reading about the genetic mechanisms involved in the process of conception, couples can appreciate the reasons conception may take longer and be more difficult than anticipated. Since genetic abnormalities normally occur in embryos with such high frequency, even if all the steps in the process of conception are perfectly aligned a pregnancy will not be produced in the vast majority of cycles, even under the most ideal of circumstances. Understanding this information is critical for several reasons. First, since complex genetic mechanisms ultimately determine when and if conception will occur, couples can more readily accept the fact that the process of conception is beyond their control. As such, they can absolve themselves of the guilt that normally plagues infertile couples. Moreover, by accepting the fact that Nature ultimately controls the process of conception through natural selection, couples will experience less emotional pain and frustration each month that pregnancy does not occur. Instead of perceiving that the failure of pregnancy to occur means that "something is wrong with them," they will understand that the embryo produced in that particular month was not destined to become a healthy baby because of genetic imperfections contained within it. In effect, the fact that Nature prevented the continued growth of a genetically flawed embryo spared the couple from giving birth to an abnormal baby.

This knowledge is also important for all couples trying to conceive since unless there is an *obvious* problem such as blocked Fallopian tubes or a very low sperm count, it will be impossible to pinpoint diagnostically where the problem may lie. More often than not, there is no problem other than Nature protecting a couple from having an abnormal baby. When we become obsessed with finding answers to unanswerable questions, anguish and frustration inevitably result.

To better cope with the pain of infertility, I advise patients to view infertility from a Zen point of view. We must learn to accept that the vast majority of questions relating to the reasons for the failure of conception are unanswerable. Because conception is a natural process, and is governed by the laws of Nature, we must learn to trust in Nature and accept its judgment as to whether an embryo is genetically perfect enough to develop into a healthy baby. Once infertile couples take that step, they will feel emotionally liberated by the knowledge that conception is a natural phenomenon, which is, for the most part, beyond human control.

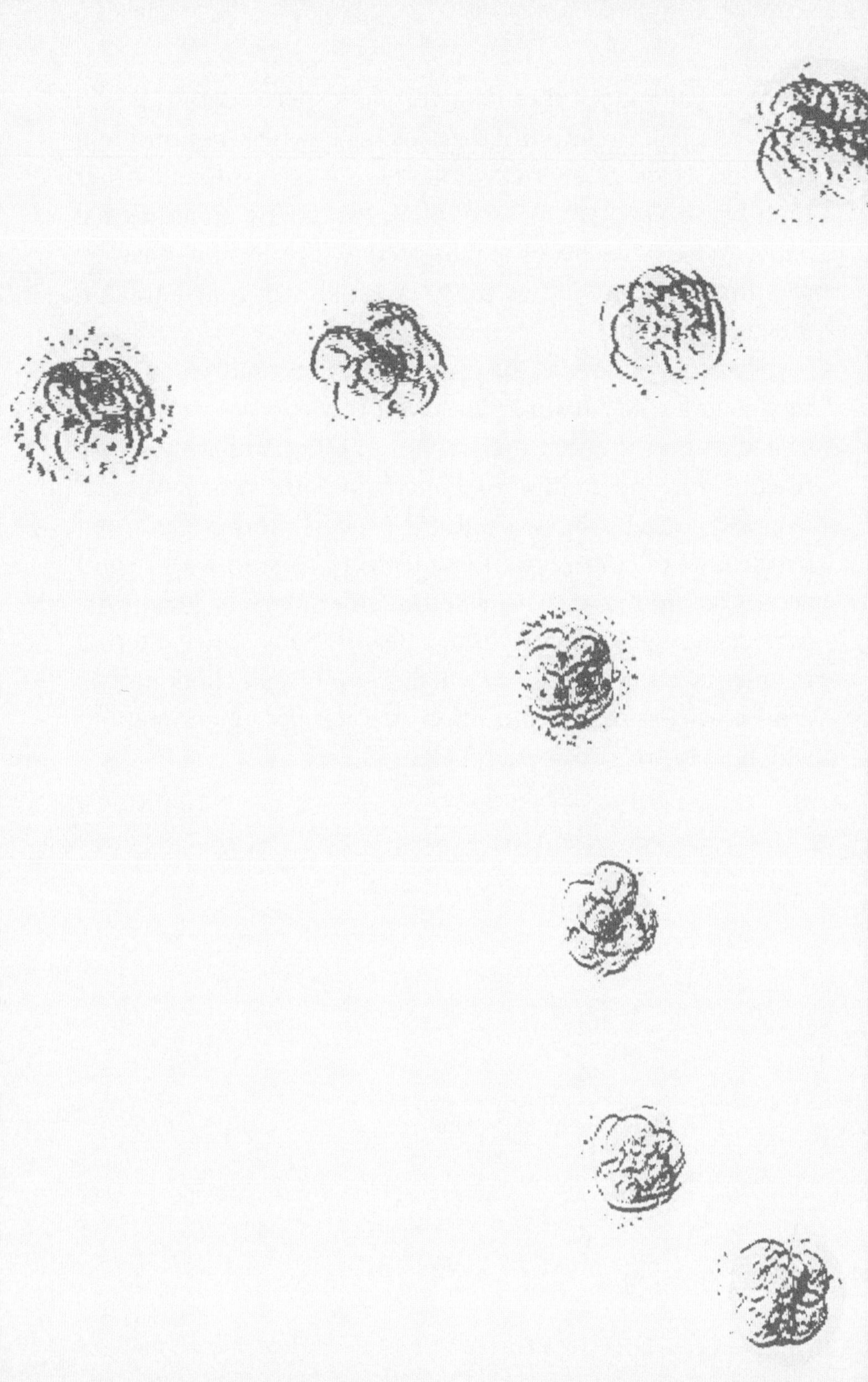

CHAPTER 3

MEDICAL APPROACHES TO INFERTILITY:

Success-oriented vs. Diagnosis-oriented

In 1996, when the first edition of the *Pregnancy Prescription* was written, the conventional medical approach to the diagnosis and treatment of infertility was far different than it is today. Prior to the early 1990s, most doctors approached infertility as if it were a disease. In the proper treatment of any illness, a competent physician does not merely prescribe treatment for a patient's symptoms. Rather, a doctor is trained to approach a patient's symptoms scientifically, through the analysis of the results of his or her medical history, physical examination and diagnostic tests. This process is meant to lead to a diagnosis. Once the diagnosis is made, an appropriate treatment can be rendered. Since involuntary infertility was once considered to be a physiological abnormality, it was treated as if it were a disease and was approached by employing the standard medical methodology deemed appropriate for treating any illness. Based on what was known about human reproduction at the time, physicians believed that the failure to conceive resulted from an anatomic or physiologic abnormality that prevented the egg and the sperm from uniting.

Before *In Vitro* Fertilization (IVF) was accepted as a "non-experimental" procedure, our knowledge of human reproduction was mainly based on observation of animal reproduction. As a result of the way scientists found that rabbits and mice reproduced, some serious misconceptions emerged. The major error of both medical professionals and the general public was that each time an egg and a sperm united, a pregnancy would result. On a month that pregnancy did not occur, the failure of conception was believed to be the result of the egg and sperm not getting together. Therefore, doctors focused almost exclusively on finding any anatomic or physiologic abnormalities that would potentially prevent a sperm and an egg from uniting. Treatment was withheld until testing revealed an abnormality thought to be the causative factor for that problem. Only then would treatment, based on the diagnosis, be initiated. While this approach is good medical practice for treating medical illnesses, we now know that it has limited applicability to infertility, since the inability to conceive is not a disease.

Our current understanding of the nature of human reproduction is a result of information obtained from the analysis of many IVF treatment cycles. The use of IVF enabled the detailed observation of the cellular events involved in the process of human fertilization and embryo growth. These were both essential parts of the conception process that could not be observed previously. It quickly became apparent that relatively few embryos actually become clinical pregnancies. Therefore, the joining of the egg and the sperm was not *the* major event to result in a pregnancy. Other, more complex factors were involved in conception. From this point, it was necessary to challenge the traditionally held beliefs about conception and to begin revising the way in which we, as physicians, diagnosed and treated infertile couples.

The Two Approaches

Any infertility specialist will want to help you conceive a child, but they all won't necessarily go about it in the same way. The differences lie in the diagnostic tests they order and in their clinical approach to your treatment. In general, infertility specialists can be considered either "diagnosis-oriented" or "success-oriented." Here, briefly, are the differences between the two approaches.

	SUCCESS-ORIENTED APPROACH	DIAGNOSIS-ORIENTED APPROACH
DIAGNOSIS	The female evaluation is based on hormonal blood tests and ultrasound examination of the reproductive organs. The male testing is a semen analysis and post-coital test. All tests are noninvasive and usually painless, and can be performed in one menstrual cycle.	The diagnostic workup includes invasive tests such as laparoscopic examination of the female reproductive organs and an endometrial biopsy, in addition to the tests conducted in the success-oriented approach. Male testing will include esoteric and costly tests for antisperm antibodies and sperm function, as well as semen analysis. Testing may take three or more months.
TREATMENT	Augmenting nature by using fertility drugs to make several eggs and placing sperm in closer proximity to them. Or, by bypassing all steps of the fertilization process that occur in the body (that may be undetectable diagnostically) that block the process of conception.	Treat diagnosed disorders and then try for natural conception. Surgical treatment may be recommended prior to less invasive forms of therapy. Allowing six or more months for natural conception to occur after corrective treatment.
IVF	May be recommended early in the process for diagnosis and treatment.	Used as a last-resort treatment option, when all other options have proved unsuccessful.

THE TRADITIONAL DIAGNOSIS-ORIENTED APPROACH

For diagnosis-oriented physicians, the primary objectives are to diagnose scientifically the cause of the couple's infertility, and then try to resolve their problem(s), so that, theoretically, the couple can conceive naturally.

Diagnosis-oriented physicians have traditionally viewed infertility as a disease. They use comprehensive diagnostic testing to determine exactly which element in a couple's reproductive process is not working properly. If the results of any of these tests signal a problem, the diagnosis-oriented physician will treat whichever problem is found. The couple will then spend several months trying to conceive on their own. If the identified problem turns out to be the only factor impeding conception, the couple will probably conceive quickly. But if the woman still does not become pregnant, it could mean that the diagnosis was incorrect, the treatment was ineffective, or there is more than one problem preventing conception. For example, the woman's age may be a coexisting problem, in addition to a single blocked Fallopian tube. Surgically repairing the blocked tube would not address the egg-quality issue related to the woman's age.

The majority of diagnosis-oriented physicians believe that advanced reproductive techniques such as IVF are treatment tools to be used only after all attempts to diagnose and correct the source of the problem have failed to help the couple conceive. In their opinion, IVF is viewed as the last resort.

THE CURRENT SUCCESS-ORIENTED APPROACH

Success-oriented physicians also believe that conception is the single most important goal of infertility treatment. These doctors feel that the best way to help an infertile couple is to perform only those diagnostic tests that will identify the major block in the reproductive process that is most likely causing the problem, then to use an appropriate treatment modality to bypass the blocked point. ***These physicians believe that infertility is not a disease, but rather a biological function involving the genetic composition of an embryo and the process of natural selection. The process of natural selection is a phenomenon that occurs in all species and ensures the birth of healthy offspring.*** Since the kinds of problems that cause infertility have no bearing on an individual's overall health nor does ill health inevitably affect fertility, success-oriented physicians believe that a diagnosis-oriented approach will not be as effective in resolving infertility as it is in treating true illnesses or injuries.

The main steps in the success-oriented approach, as described in *The Pregnancy Prescription,* are:

Step 1: The Streamlined Workup

A basic diagnostic workup consists of hormonal testing of FSH, LH, estradiol, prolactin and thyroid. It also includes a sonogram to check for ovarian reserve and endometriosis in the ovaries, as well as the identification of any potential abnormalities of the uterus. The evaluation is best performed on cycle day 2-4, during the menstrual period. After the period is over, a hydrosonogram is performed to ensure that the Fallopian tubes are open and that there are no fibroids or polyps inside the cavity of the uterus. Then, at the time of anticipated ovulation, a post-coital test and another sonogram to document that an egg follicle is actually present, are performed. This diagnostic evaluation is rapid and involves no painful or invasive procedures. Most significantly, it demonstrates whether the couple is potentially fertile or, if not, which factors are most likely preventing them from conceiving.

Step 2: Clomiphene Citrate and Intrauterine Insemination (IUI)

The oral fertility drug, clomiphene citrate (brand names Clomid™, Serophene™), is used to increase the number of eggs the woman is able to produce. Intrauterine insemination, which calls for a specially prepared sperm specimen to be inserted into the top of the woman's uterus, provides the sperm with direct access to the Fallopian tubes, bypassing possible problems in the vagina and cervix.

Step 3: Gonadotropins and Intrauterine Insemination (IUI)

Injectable fertility drugs (gonadotropins: Bravelle™, Menopur™, Follistim™ and Gonal F™) usually induce the woman to produce far greater numbers of mature eggs (controlled ovarian hyperstimulation) than the oral fertility medications used in Step 2. This is combined with IUI to ensure that enough sperm are in proximity to the multiple eggs that have been produced.

Step 4: *In Vitro* Fertilization (IVF)
In IVF, the eggs are removed from the ovary and fertilized in the laboratory away from any potentially detrimental factors within the woman's body. The resulting embryos are placed back into the uterus. The embryologist may use Intracytoplasmic Sperm Injection (ICSI), in which a single sperm is injected into the egg, to help the fertilization process along.

Step 5: IVF with Donor Eggs
When a woman's egg supply is found to be either depleted or unable to be fertilized, her partner's sperm may be used to fertilize donor eggs. The resulting embryos are placed back into the woman's uterus and, should she become pregnant, the baby will be her biological—if not genetic—offspring.

After the workup has been completed, the starting point of treatment is determined by both the diagnostic workup and the couple's wishes. If a couple has a long-standing history of infertility, they could have the choice of starting at step 2, step 3 or step 4. To define more precisely the best initial therapy, factors such as the patient's age and the post-coital test must be considered. If the woman is 40 years old with a normal workup and low ovarian reserve, IUI would not be beneficial since the PCT was normal. Nor would IVF be the ideal treatment choice since her low ovarian reserve suggests an oocyte quality problem, which is not treatable with IVF. In this case, pregnancy, if it occurs, will happen either naturally or with the use of donor oocytes. However, many couples in this situation will want to try an IVF cycle in the hope that they will be one of the few who will beat the odds prior to moving on to step 5. Yet if a woman is under 32 years of age with a long history of infertility and good ovarian reserve, IVF is a reasonable starting point.

Former infertility patients confirm that the success-oriented approach is much easier from an emotional perspective. From a patient's point of view, any time not spent in the direct pursuit of pregnancy is time wasted. Months lost to testing, aimless "trying" and prescribed time off can cause anguish to a woman who wants nothing more than a new life in her belly. The beauty of the success-oriented approach is that conception is possible within one month from the initial consultation.

Although success-oriented physicians don't believe that all advanced reproductive techniques (like IVF) are right for each and every patient, they do maintain that, for many couples, IVF can increase a couple's chances of conceiving *more quickly and cost effectively* by:

- **Eliminating** the need for some of the more expensive, invasive and time-consuming diagnostic tests
- **Identifying** otherwise undetectable problems that are most likely preventing the couple from conceiving
- **Bypassing** the steps that appear most likely to be causing the couple's infertility

- **Offering a significant chance of conception every time it is performed** by bringing egg and sperm together in an environment that provides optimum conditions for fertilization and embryo development

HYPOTHETICAL CLINICAL CASE STUDIES

Here are two scenarios that illustrate how the course of treatment of the same couple would differ if they consulted both a diagnosis-oriented and a success-oriented specialist. Let's call the couples Susan and Mark and Kate and Steven. Their clinical histories are very typical and representative of many couples that I have treated in the past. I have crafted these theoretic case studies to illustrate the possible differences in the two types of treatment approaches and how they might affect the couples' therapy.

SUSAN AND MARK— THE SUCCESS-ORIENTED APPROACH

Susan and Mark, both 36-year-old lawyers, had been unsuccessfully trying to conceive on their own for six months. Susan had an early, uncomplicated abortion before she met Mark, and the couple had been lax in practicing birth control for several years before they started trying for a pregnancy.

Although nothing suspicious was noted during her case history, Susan's blood tested positive for anti-chlamydia antibodies, indicating that she had previously been infected by that organism.

Because he suspected that Susan's tubes might have been damaged as a result of the infection, the doctor recommended that she undergo a hydrosonogram. The results showed that one tube was completely blocked, but the other tube was open.

Since Susan had tested positive for a previous chlamydia infection, had been unable to become pregnant on her own and was known to have at least one damaged tube, the doctor suspected that the other tube might have been compromised as well. Taking Susan's age into account, he recommended that the couple proceed directly to an IVF cycle, which would both bypass the tubes and enable the doctor to determine whether there might also be a fertilization problem or another issue with Mark's sperm.

With medication, Susan produced only six eggs for the IVF cycle—four of which were successfully fertilized by Mark's sperm. Although the couple elected to have all four embryos transferred back into Susan's uterus, she did not conceive during that cycle. The doctor suspected that two concurrent problems were causing Susan's infertility: the problem with her tubes and possible effects of age on her oocytes. Since they had achieved good fertilization, the doctor encouraged Susan and Mark to continue with IVF treatment.

SUSAN AND MARK—THE DIAGNOSIS-ORIENTED APPROACH

Let's see what might have happened if Susan and Mark had consulted a diagnosis-oriented fertility specialist.

The results of the cervical cultures normally performed during a standard workup would have been negative for Susan, since she wasn't currently suffering from the chlamydia infection. Therefore, unless the doctor performed a blood test for anti-chlamydia antibodies, he might not have thought to have Susan undergo a hysterosalpingogram (HSG) so early in the diagnostic process. Instead, he might have sent her home with urine testing kits to monitor her ovulation and instructions as to how to schedule intercourse for the appropriate time after the LH surge. At the same time,

Mark would have been asked to undergo a semen analysis, the results of which would be normal.

After a few cycles of supposedly normal ovulation but no resulting conception, the doctor would then have been likely to suggest an HSG. Since the x-rays showed a blockage in one Fallopian tube, the doctor would have performed a laparoscopy, using surgery both to repair the known blockage and to look for endometriosis or another anatomical problem that might be keeping Susan from conceiving. Although the operation would be performed on an outpatient basis, Susan would need to undergo general anesthesia during the procedure and she would experience pain and soreness for some days afterward.

After her laparoscopy, Susan (her damaged tube newly unblocked) and Mark would be ready to try again. If pregnancy did not occur after three or four more months of trying naturally, the doctor might help things along with fertility drugs and inseminations. Unfortunately, Susan would still not become pregnant. The doctor might perform a second HSG to make sure her tubes hadn't closed up again, or he might order additional tests both for her (an endometrial biopsy) and for Mark (hamster egg penetration test). None of these tests would reveal what was preventing the pregnancy.

Finally, the doctor might throw up his hands and suggest that the couple try IVF as a last resort. Why? Because in addition to the blockage of the distal (outer) end of one of her Fallopian tubes, Susan's infection had also caused subtle damage to the insides of both tubes. The damage was both *undetectable and untreatable.* So although the surgery eliminated Susan's most obvious physical problem, she was still incapable of conceiving naturally. IVF offered her the only genuine chance for a pregnancy.

KATE AND STEVEN—
THE SUCCESS-ORIENTED APPROACH

Kate, an artist, and Steven, a writer, had been trying to conceive for nearly two years. Since Kate was only 31-years-old, the couple was reluctant to consult a fertility specialist, but since both wanted a big family, they decided that it would be wise to seek help.

Neither case history indicated any problem. Kate's hydrosonogram and blood tests were normal. However, Steven's semen analysis showed that his sperm had marginally abnormal morphology (shape) and motility (movement). A physical exam revealed that he suffered from a varicocele (varicose vein of the testes).

The doctor recommended a diagnostic IVF cycle to determine whether Steven's sperm were capable of fertilizing Kate's eggs. Thanks to medication, Kate produced 12 eggs, which the embryologist divided into two groups. He exposed the first group to Steven's sperm in the normal manner to determine whether they could fertilize naturally and performed ICSI (injection of a single sperm directly into the egg) with the eggs in the second group. Two of the eggs in the first group fertilized, as did five from the ICSI group. Unfortunately, none of the four embryos that were transferred back to Kate's uterus implanted; neither did the remaining three embryos, which had been frozen and then thawed and transferred into her uterus during a subsequent cycle.

For their next IVF cycle, Kate was able to produce only nine eggs. Thanks to ICSI, Steven's sperm successfully fertilized six of the eggs *in vitro*. The couple elected to transfer all six embryos back into Kate's uterus. Several weeks later, Kate learned she was pregnant with twins. Steven's varicocele and marginally abnormal sperm had appeared to be the obvious cause of this couple's infertility. But the initial IVF trial demonstrated that, even unassisted, Steven's sperm were capable of fertilizing some of Kate's eggs, but at a lower percentage rate than normal. Their inability to conceive was possibly caused by two factors: a reduced fertilization rate combined with a genetically based embryo quality issue that was successfully resolved by the IVF procedure.

KATE AND STEVEN— THE DIAGNOSIS-ORIENTED APPROACH

As soon as a diagnosis-oriented physician would have become aware of Steven's sperm abnormalities (abnormal shape and movement), he would have suspected a varicocele. When the physical exam confirmed his suspicions, the doctor would have recommended that Steven undergo surgery to correct the problem—especially since the results of the couple's complete diagnostic workup would have revealed no other problems that could be causing their infertility.

The operation, though not serious, would have caused Steven some discomfort for several weeks. A post-surgical semen analysis would probably have demonstrated some improvement in his sperms' motility and morphology, but the change would not be dramatic. One year later, Kate still would not have become pregnant. The doctor would probably have advised the couple to try fertility drugs combined with intrauterine insemination, since he could find no treatable cause for their continued inability to conceive. He would advise them to proceed to IVF only after it had become clear that the IUI was not succeeding.

POTENTIAL PITFALLS OF THE DIAGNOSIS-ORIENTED APPROACH

Both of these case studies indicate that a problem with the diagnosis-oriented approach is that many of the diagnostic techniques and procedures traditionally used to treat infertility can be painful, unreliable, invasive and time consuming. This is an especially important consideration for women in their mid-to-late 30s and early 40s, who are at the mercy of their biological clocks.

But perhaps more important, the case studies illustrate that many of the factors responsible for causing infertility are impossible to diagnose accurately by any method. To complicate matters, several causative factors may exist simultaneously. The American Society for Reproductive Medicine estimates that fewer than half of all infertile couples can be helped by techniques such as fertility drugs, simple inseminations and surgery. In addition, there may be more than one factor preventing the couple from conceiving. It may be possible to cure one problem, but other undiagnosed factors could still make unassisted conception impossible.

The reality is that the process of conception is too complex to allow for the diagnosis and treatment of all the potential factors that may be causing a couple's infertility. There are simply too many steps at which problems may occur, both at the microscopic and genetic level. Only the most obvious causes can be accurately diagnosed and resolved.

SO WHY ISN'T EVERYONE SUCCESS-ORIENTED?

Since the original edition of *The Pregnancy Prescription* was published ten years ago, there has been a natural evolution in the field of reproductive medicine. One of the most significant changes is that currently most reproductive endocrinologists advocate the success-oriented approach in the treatment of infertile couples. In past years, the success-oriented strategy wasn't universally embraced because it was not considered sufficiently scientific and because of its reliance on advanced reproductive techniques, such as IVF, which were fairly new at the time. Now days, most physicians and patients are likely to be better informed as to the potential value of these techniques for diagnostic as well as treatment purposes.

CONCERNS ABOUT POTENTIAL RISKS WITH FERTILITY MEDICATIONS AND IVF

In the past ten years, most physicians have been able to gain enough experience with IVF to see that it is a minimally invasive, brief, outpatient procedure, which entails only a small degree of discomfort and risk for the vast majority of patients. In addition, statistics from thousands of IVF cycles document that the egg retrieval procedure has an extremely low rate of complications when it is performed by experienced physicians. An in depth discussion of potential complications is found in the chapter on the IVF retrieval. What also is of concern to some couples contemplating fertility enhancing therapy is the possibility that the treatments will have an adverse effect on a fetus. Please rest assured that babies born as a result of fertility treatments are no different than those conceived naturally.

Couples are also concerned about the short and long term risks associated with the use of fertility medications. The major short term risk of the injectable drugs is over-stimulation of the ovaries, resulting in a condition called the ovarian hyperstimulation syndrome. Fortunately, most women taking injectables are not at high risk for developing this syndrome. This complication is discussed in the chapter on injectable fertility medications.

A number of articles which, in the past, have appeared in the popular press claimed that the medications used in IVF may increase a woman's chances of developing ovarian cancer. The most important fact to remember is that *the major fertility medications that are used in IVF are completely natural.* They consist of FSH, LH AND HCG, which are hormones circulating, at varying levels, in every woman's body from the time of puberty until death. If these hormones were actually carcinogenic, I would imagine that a huge number of women would be stricken with ovarian cancer, which, in reality, is fortunately rare. In my experience of 30 years in a busy clinical practice, I do not recall more than three cases of this malignancy, and none of these cases occurred in women who were treated with fertility drugs. Rather, ovarian cancer may be related to a genetic (familial) factor, possibly in association with a gene that causes a high incidence of breast cancer in certain families. Also of significance is a statistical association between ovarian cancer and nulliparity (never having been pregnant). Finally, the general consensus on this issue by the American Society of Reproductive Medicine, having reviewed all existing studies on the relationship of fertility drugs and ovarian cancer, is that fertility drugs are not implicated as a causative factor in any form of cancer.

There are some data suggesting that women who have taken the fertility drug clomid for more than 12 cycles may have a slightly higher incidence of ovarian cancer than would be expected. Since women currently rarely take clomid for more than three or four cycles, this factoid should be of no concern. What the public may not understand is that many experts consider the study, on which that charge was based, to have been poorly designed. Actually, ovarian cancer is related to nulliparity (never having been pregnant) rather than to the drugs used to treat infertility.

CONFUSING SUCCESS RATES

There is much confusion about the rates of conception resulting from infertility treatments. Whether a couple will ultimately conceive will largely depend upon several key factors, all of which are beyond human control. These include a woman's age, her egg reserve, the quality of her partner's sperm, and the genetic content of the embryos produced. The most important factor of all is the genetic quality of the embryos produced. If an embryo is genetically imperfect, it cannot develop into a perfectly healthy baby. This is Nature's failsafe mechanism for preventing the birth of unhealthy or otherwise imperfect offspring. This phenomenon occurs in all species and is known as natural selection. Natural selection operates at the genetic level. Since the process of fertilization is so complex at the genetic level, the majority of embryos produced from eggs of excellent quality will be genetically imperfect. Understanding this phenomenon explains why, despite transferring the most perfect appearing embryos into the uterus, pregnancy will not occur 100% of the time, as would be expected logically. Rather, because of the high rate of genetic imperfections normally found in embryos, pregnancy can only be expected to occur, at best, 35% of the time.

COST MISPERCEPTIONS

IVF is perceived as being extremely expensive. However, although the cost of an IVF procedure in the US can range from $6,000 to $15,000, this figure can vary significantly according to geographic location and individual clinic. Although some clinics are at the higher end of the scale, now many clinics offer fees that are at the lower end of the spectrum. Thorough investigation of all costs and fees should be completed prior to undergoing treatment. Fortunately, some insurance companies pay for a limited number of IVF cycles. It is therefore advisable to obtain a health insurance policy that includes an infertility rider, providing coverage for fertility treatments.

SUMMARY

All fields of medicine are in a constant state of evolution as physicians integrate new technology into the way they treat their patients. As they become more comfortable with the new technologies, their practices usually change. Such is the case in reproductive medicine. As doctors treating infertile couples gained more experience with IVF they became more aware of its treatment potential, especially in cases in which there may be no diagnosable condition present that could be causing infertility. Consequently, most infertility specialists have abandoned the traditional diagnostic-oriented approach and have become more success-oriented. The realization that infertility is not a disease, but rather a result of the forces of natural selection, makes it exempt from the diagnostic orientation that is mandatory for the highest standard of medical practice in most other specialties. From speaking to many colleagues in the field, I find that most infertility doctors now believe good medical practice is compatible with eliminating extensive diagnostic testing and seek to employ more empiric treatments that can expand the power of nature and help many couples conceive more quickly and cost effectively.

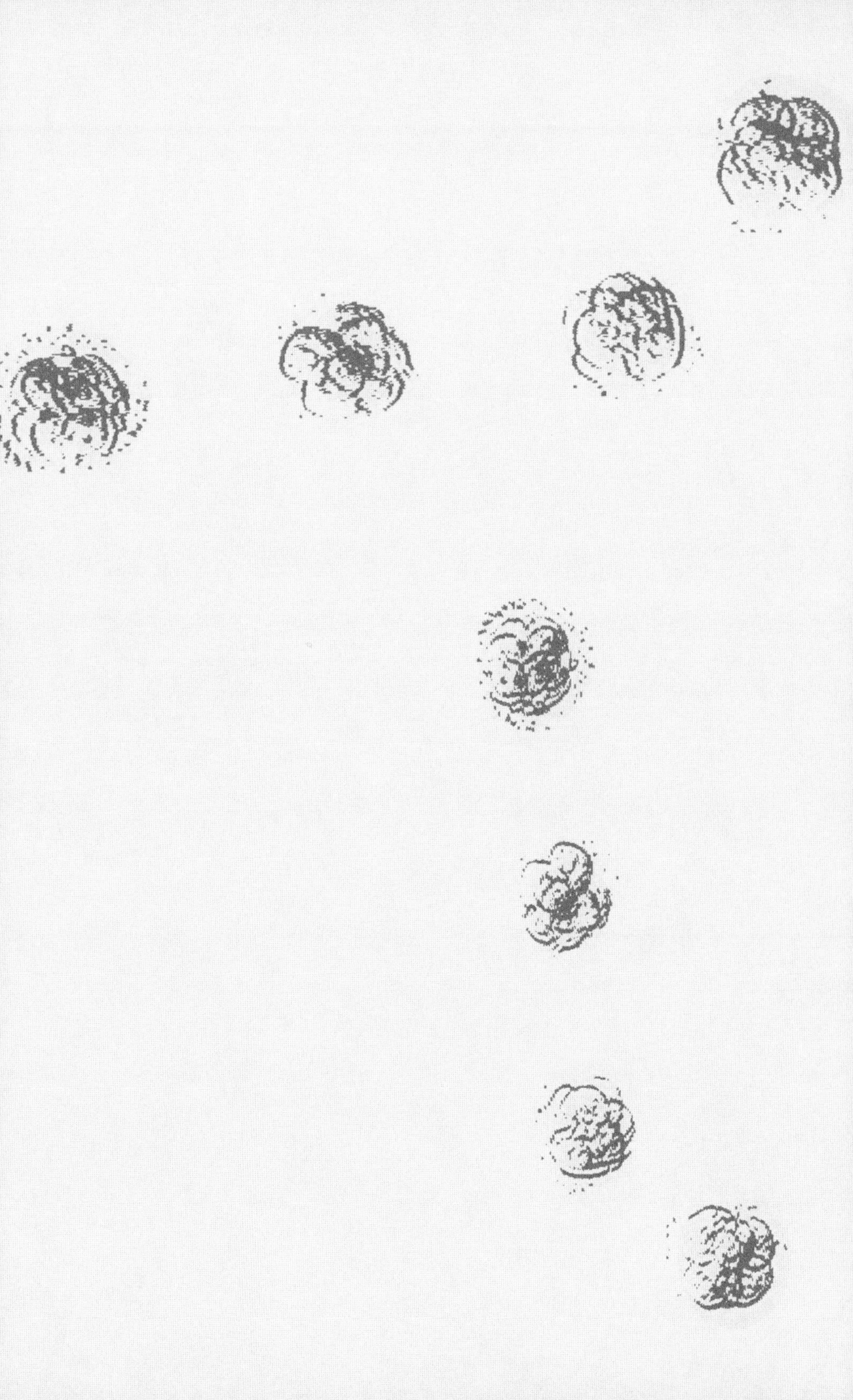

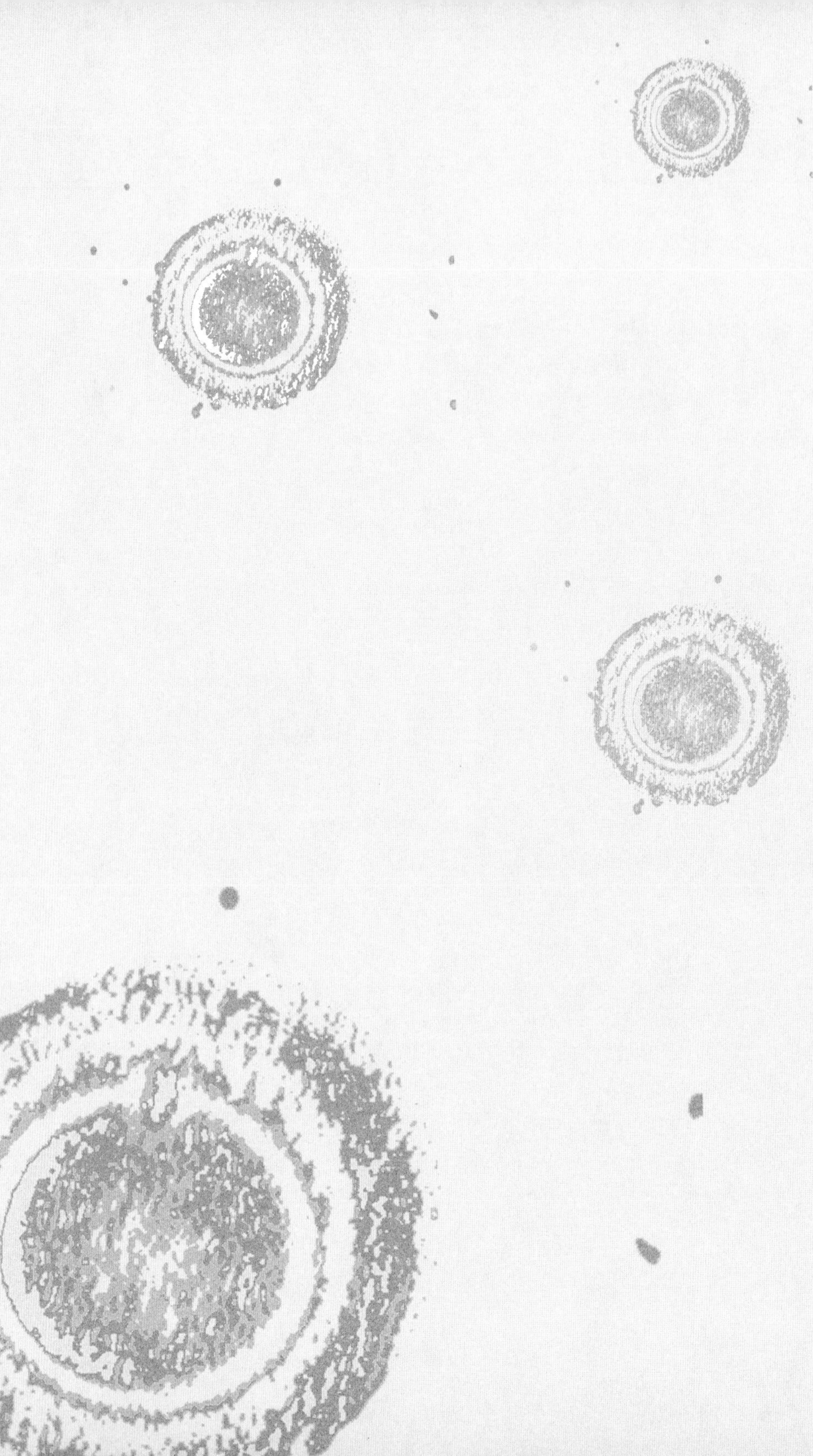

CHAPTER 4

A STREAMLINED EVALUATION OF FERTILITY POTENTIAL:

What Fertility Tests Are Needed and What Their Results Mean to You

The first step for you and your partner in investigating your fertility issues is to undergo a diagnostic workup. The number of tests that you are advised to undergo and the amount of that time you spend on testing, rather than treatment, will largely depend on whether your doctor follows a diagnosis- or success-oriented approach to infertility treatment. In this chapter, the difference between the two approaches will be illustrated. In this way, you, as a patient, will thoroughly understand the various diagnostic tests that may be recommended, as well as their relevance and significance.

Even if your doctor advises only a few of the most basic infertility tests, you may find some portions of the workup embarrassing, or feel that your privacy is being invaded. You will probably need to answer detailed questions about your sexual practices. Women may find themselves lying on an examination table with their legs spread more often than they would have ever thought possible! Their partners will probably become adept at ejaculating into sterile containers.

Distasteful as all this may be, don't let shyness deter you from your goal of conceiving a child. Your doctor and the rest of the office staff should try to make you feel as comfortable as possible with whatever testing or treatments need to be done. They will be scrupulous about protecting your privacy, as patients' confidentiality is protected by federal laws.

THE DIAGNOSIS-ORIENTED WORKUP

Diagnosis-oriented fertility specialists use tests and procedures to determine which parts of their patients' reproductive systems aren't working correctly. Their meticulous and exhaustive testing will include many—if not all—of the following:

THE DIAGNOSIS-ORIENTED WORKUP FOR HER

- Patient history
- Physical exam
- Cervical cultures to test for current infection by chlamydia or mycoplasma
- Blood tests for hormone levels: FSH, LH, estradiol, prolactin, thyroid
- Blood test for Inhibin "B," a hormone secreted by the ovaries
- Ovulation tests via basal body temperature reporting or at-home urine testing kits
- Pelvic sonogram
- At least one hysterosalpingogram (HSG): a dye-assisted x-ray of the woman's uterus and Fallopian tubes
- At least one post-coital test (PCT) near the time of ovulation: after the couple has intercourse, the doctor examines the woman's cervical mucus under a microscope to evaluate whether her partner's sperm can function inside of her
- An endometrial biopsy: the doctor removes a sample of the woman's uterine lining and sends it to a pathologist for analysis
- At least one diagnostic/therapeutic laparoscopy: a surgical procedure that allows the doctor to view the woman's internal organs

THE DIAGNOSIS-ORIENTED WORKUP FOR HIM

- Patient history
- Physical exam
- At least one semen analysis
- A hamster test to determine whether the sperm is able to penetrate a hamster egg
- Sperm DNA fragmentation testing

THE DIAGNOSIS-ORIENTED WORKUP FOR BOTH

- Anti-sperm antibody blood tests to determine whether either partner is producing substances that may block fertilization of an egg

THE SUCCESS-ORIENTED WORKUP

Success-oriented physicians need to learn enough from the workup to determine which form of treatment to start with. They tend to rely on a few rapid, basic, non-invasive tests to rule out major and obvious problems. ***Success-oriented physicians believe that the majority of disorders that cause infertility are most often impossible to diagnose accurately, as the problems occur on a cellular or microscopic level.*** This means that all but the most obvious defects that are responsible for the failure of conception are below the threshold of detection of traditional diagnostic tests. For success-oriented infertility specialists, *In Vitro* Fertilization (IVF) is the most valuable diagnostic and therapeutic tool available.

The success-oriented, streamlined workup can save you precious time (the complete battery of standard infertility tests can take up to a year or longer) and pain (some standard diagnostic tests involve surgery). They can also substantially reduce the costs normally associated with the traditional diagnostic and therapeutic process.

THE SUCCESS-ORIENTED WORKUP FOR HER

PATIENT HISTORY

Health and reproductive histories are important elements of a streamlined workup. The information provided during a patient history can help the doctor decide whether the couple should proceed directly to an IVF trial or if other tests and/or procedures should be performed first.

Age

First and foremost, the doctor needs to know the patient's age. In general, the younger the woman, the better her chances for conceiving, since the quality of a woman's eggs tends to decline as she gets older. For example, if a 37- to 42-year-old woman has been able to conceive easily in the past but her two most recent conceptions ended in early miscarriage, it would be reasonable to assume that her eggs have been adversely affected by her age. The doctor would probably perform hormonal tests and evaluate her ovarian reserve to verify this hypothesis; however, such a patient could prove infertile despite normal test values.

Medical History

Since certain diseases, such as rheumatoid arthritis, may affect a woman's ability to maintain a pregnancy, the doctor needs to know the patient's complete medical history. Information about her menstrual periods—their regularity, duration, heaviness of flow, etc.—as well as any previous gynecologic infections and/or surgery is also vital. It is particularly important to know if a patient has had any abortions, since any surgical procedure, whether major or minor, may result in subtle, undetectable tubal damage or in the formation of internal scar tissue.

Reproductive History

A couple's reproductive history is critical to a physician, since it may suggest the most likely place to begin the diagnostic evaluation. Although it may be embarrassing to admit to having had a sexually transmitted disease or an abortion in the past, it is imperative that your doctor be aware of it. (If you cannot discuss this type of information in front of your spouse, you can easily arrange a private meeting with your doctor, who will indicate in your medical records that the information is to be held in strict confidence.) Having such a reproductive history would suggest to a physician that he or she should begin the patient's evaluation with a test to see if the Fallopian tubes are open and a blood test for anti-chlamydia antibodies. The doctor also needs to know whether the patient has ever been pregnant. A previous pregnancy in a woman who is under the age of 35 is usually considered a good sign, since it suggests that she was born with an egg supply that is of good genetic quality. However, if a woman with normal menstrual periods and patent (open) tubes has never conceived despite unprotected intercourse with several partners over a period of years, her history strongly suggests "unexplained infertility." Such patients present a difficult diagnostic challenge, since the factors causing their infertility are beyond the scope of currently used diagnostic tests. As such, time should not be wasted with further testing, observation, or any treatment other than IVF. Since the majority of patients with unexplained infertility have fertilization failure or egg and embryo quality issues, an IVF trial gives the physician an opportunity to determine the most likely cause of her failure to conceive—and affords the patient an opportunity to achieve a pregnancy at the same time.

PELVIC SONOGRAM

A pelvic sonogram is the most important examination for infertile women. To perform the sonogram, a technician or physician inserts a small probe that is shaped like a wand into the woman's vagina. Although some women find the procedure a little embarrassing the first few times it is performed, a vaginal ultrasound exam is painless. And unlike abdominal sonograms, this exam does not require the patient to have a full bladder.

The sonographic image projected onto the screen shows the size and shape of the uterus and endometrial cavity, as well as the presence and position of the ovaries. It also indicates whether there is a reserve of eggs present in the ovaries. This is the most important part of the evaluation, since the greater the supply of eggs in the ovaries, the better the woman's chance of becoming pregnant. This ovarian reserve is also predictive of how well a woman will respond to fertility medications. Women with larger numbers of eggs in their ovaries will produce more eggs in response to fertility-enhancing drugs. In addition, the ovarian reserve is important in helping the physician determine which fertility drug regimen is the most effective treatment for a particular patient. Finally, if there is low ovarian reserve, the physician can determine the cause of infertility. Usually, when relatively few resting egg follicles remain, those eggs are the most genetically compromised. It should be noted, however, that the determination of egg reserve is entirely subjective and depends on the experience and expertise of the sonographer and physician, as well as on the age and the clinical history of the woman.

A sonogram can detect abnormalities in the uterus and ovaries and show the physician if the Fallopian tubes are swollen or filled with fluid (hydrosalpinx), which means that they were probably blocked as a result of a prior tubal infection. It can also detect endometrial cysts (endometrosis) inside the ovaries, which cannot be visualized by other methods (including laparoscopy). Such cysts could explain the cause of infertility, since endometriosis adversely affects both egg production and quality.

Ultrasound also enables the physician to visualize the interior of the uterus and determine the quality of the lining, which is where the pregnancy implants and develops. Pathologic conditions of the uterus that may have a negative impact on conception, such as leiomyomas (fibroids) and adenomyosis (endometrial tissue growing abnormally in the muscular walls of the uterus), can be detected via ultrasound.

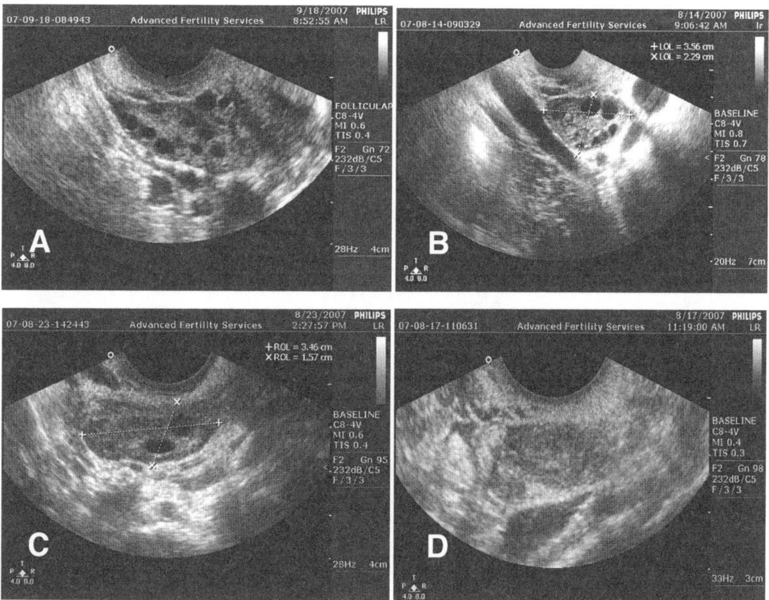

Fig. 1. A. ***Sonogram showing an ovary with good egg reserve.***
B. ***Sonogram showing an ovary with moderate egg reserve.***
C. ***Sonogram showing an ovary with low egg reserve.***
D. ***Sonogram showing a menopausal ovary.***

TESTS FOR INFECTION

Although vaginal infections do not cause infertility, pelvic infections caused by certain organisms, such as chlamydia, can result in irreparable damage to the Fallopian tubes and prevent a woman from being able to conceive naturally. This can happen in one of two ways: either the tubes become occluded (blocked) as a result of an inflammatory response to the infection or the tubal lining becomes damaged, thereby interfering with its ability to propel the oocyte (egg) or embryo towards the uterus.

Since chlamydia infections do not always cause symptoms, a woman may not know if she has ever been infected; the only way to be sure is to test the blood for the presence of the anti-chlamydial antibody. If the test results are positive, the woman may have been infected with chlamydia at least once in the (usually distant) past. It is most important to understand that a positive antibody test does not mean that the woman is currently infected or contagious. Rather, the antibodies are a clue—or fingerprint—to indicate a past exposure to the pathogen. And if that woman's tubes appear to be open and yet she has been unable to become pregnant, the infection may have caused undetectable damage to the lining of her Fallopian tubes. It is likely that such women will need to undergo IVF treatment to bypass their tubes in order to become pregnant.

Mycoplasma, another organism that has been implicated as a possible cause of infertility and miscarriage, can be difficult to detect via a culture. Therefore, at some point during their infertility treatment it may be useful for the male and the female to have simultaneous treatment with an antibiotic such as Vibramycin™ (doxycycline: a tetracycline derivative), which has proven effective against the organism. These days, such antibiotic treatment is considered as prophylactic prior to the egg retrieval in IVF. Hypothetically, the antibiotic "sterilizes" the female reproductive tract, as well as the male's seminal fluid. Side effects of the medication may include nausea, diarrhea, yeast infections and photosensitivity. To offset these potential side effects, patients that are being administered Vibramycin must take it on a full stomach. They should also eat yogurt or drink acidophyllis milk and stay out of direct sunlight while on this medication. If vaginal itching or burning results, your physician will provide a prescription for a cream or a pill to relieve this uncomfortable condition.

Some older (and largely uncorroborated) data indicate that antibiotic treatment may increase the chances for pregnancy. However, in my experience neither mycoplasma nor ureaplasma has ever been a significant factor in infertility. Patients should avoid infertility treatment that consists of intravenous or long courses of high-dose antibiotic therapy. Such treatments are ineffective and may cause serious medical complications. In fact, if such treatment is recommended, you should immediately seek a second opinion.

HORMONE LEVEL TESTING

Although the quality of a woman's eggs usually declines as she ages, chronological age is not always the best way to assess a woman's potential fertility. Hormone level testing cannot always help to predict which women will be able to conceive. However, abnormal levels of certain hormones can be reliable indicators of which women will be unable to achieve a pregnancy.

Follicle Stimulating Hormone (FSH)

As the name suggests, this is the hormone that signals the ovaries to begin producing an egg for a new cycle. Testing a woman's FSH level on day 2 to 3 of her menstrual cycle provides the best indication of how well she will respond to fertility drugs—a measure that correlates with her overall chances for becoming pregnant. Again, the test suggests whether pregnancy cannot occur rather than whether it can. In general, the lower a woman's FSH on day 2 to 3 of her cycle, the better.

FSH	CHANCES FOR PREGNANCY
<10 mlU/mL	Best chances for pregnancy
10-15 mlU/mL	May not respond well to ovarian stimulation, but pregnancy is still very possible
15-20 mlU/mL	Depleted pool of eggs; reduced chances for pregnancy
20-25 mlU/mL	May ovulate, but prognosis for pregnancy is poor
>25 mlU/mL	Will probably not become pregnant without donor eggs

Since FSH levels fluctuate on a monthly basis, the day 2 or 3 FSH level predicts a woman's ovulation response for that particular cycle only. For example, if a 40-year-old woman has an FSH level of 19 on day 3, she will probably not respond well to fertility drugs that month and it would be wise to withhold treatment for that particular cycle. During her next cycle, however, her day 3 FSH level may drop to 12, and she may be better able to respond to the medications. Unfortunately, once a woman has been shown to have a high FSH level, her chances for becoming pregnant are greatly reduced—even though she may occasionally produce numerous eggs in response to fertility drugs. An exception is the younger (28- to 35-year-old) woman who may be able to become pregnant despite an occasional "high FSH" month. In fact, in my practice, a 38-year-old woman conceived naturally during a cycle in which her FSH level was 31! Moreover, the pregnancy resulted in a healthy baby. Therefore, it is important to remember that the FSH levels are not the be all and end all! It is wise not to panic if FSH is occasionally on the high side.

The case I just described, as well as similar experiences, equally exceptional, have brought me to the humbling realization that—after treating infertile patients for 30 years—the more I learn, the less I understand. There are no "absolute truths" in the diagnosis and treatment of infertile couples. Happy exceptions occur almost as frequently as the "sure thing" treatments (there is no such thing!) that are ultimately unsuccessful.

Estradiol (Estrogen)

A woman's estradiol level on day 2 to 3 of her cycle is another important predictor of her potential fertility. If her estradiol level on day 2 to 3 is greater than 80 mg/ml, she may be experiencing abnormal follicle production—similar, in pattern, to early pre-menopause. Although this may not be a good sign for a woman who wants to become pregnant, sometimes an elevated estrogen level may be caused by a hormonally active ovarian cyst. These cysts will almost always disappear after treatment with birth control pills for three weeks.

Prolactin

Elevated prolactin (the hormone that stimulates milk secretion) levels can interfere with a doctor's ability to induce ovulation in some patients, while others who have elevated levels remain able to ovulate normally. This is because a woman can secrete any of five varieties of the prolactin hormone molecule. Although a blood test will detect elevated levels of any of these five varieties, only one or two actually affect the menstrual cycle. Elevated levels of the others may cause certain physical effects (e.g., the production of fluid from the nipples), but since they do not inhibit or block ovulation, they do not need to be treated. Women with prolactin levels that are significantly elevated should undergo a CAT scan or MRI study of their pituitary gland to determine whether a small, benign growth is causing excess production of prolactin. Normal prolactin levels range from 0 to 35. If your prolactin level is between 35 and 100, don't be too concerned about the possibility of having a brain tumor. If a pituitary growth were actually present, the prolactin level would be between 100 and 1,000. Even with very high prolactin levels associated with pituitary growths, a medication called Parlodel will quickly bring these levels into the normal range and will actually cause the tumor to shrink. Another medication, called Dostinex, has also been used successfully to treat elevated prolactin levels with a once-weekly dosage; however, recent studies suggest the possibility of rare, but potentially serious side effects. Until this issue is clarified, it is wise to use Parlodel. Surgery is rarely, if ever, required to treat pituitary gland growths.

Elevations in prolactin levels may also be caused by an under-active thyroid gland—a condition called hypothyroidism (see the following section). The thyroid gland controls the body's metabolism. Menstrual irregularities and lack of normal ovulation in patients with an under-active thyroid may be caused by elevations in prolactin levels. Therefore, both the thyroid hormone as well as levels of prolactin should be measured in all infertile females, especially in those with irregular menstrual periods, unexplained weight gain or unusual fatigue. Elevated prolactin levels in males may cause impotence or very low sexual drive.

The Thyroid Gland

From the 1940s to the 1960s, many infertile women, as well as those with a history of recurrent miscarriage, were treated empirically (without laboratory tests, but having the clinical symptoms associated with an underactive thyroid gland) with thyroid medication. From a purely "scientific" point of view, most doctors believe that only severely underactive thyroid function (defined as elevated TSH and low levels of thyroid hormones) that interferes with the menstrual cycle—by either stopping menstruation or interfering with ovulation—causes infertility. However, there is a subgroup of women that experience the typical symptoms of an underactive thyroid gland but whose thyroid function tests are within the lower part of the normal range. These patients have what I call "subclinical hypothyroidism." The symptoms of this condition may include fatigue, feeling cold, water retention and an inability to lose weight. The hair and skin may be unusually dry and the fingernails brittle. There is also frequently a history of hypothyroidism in the patient's family—mother, sisters or maternal aunts. A simple "old fashioned" way to measure thyroid function is to have such a patient take her oral temperature before getting out of bed in the morning, starting on day 1 of her period and continuing up to the point of ovulation. (Remember that body temperature rises by one degree after ovulation.) If during this time period the woman's oral temperature reads consistently at less than 97.5 degrees Fahrenheit, she is considered to have subclinical hypothyroidism. Her low basal body temperature is a sign of a slow (cold) metabolism, much like a car engine that runs cold when it cannot get enough gas. In most cases, these patients will improve symptomatically when given thyroid hormone supplementation. They will feel more energetic, lose weight, feel less cold, and see improvements in their skin and hair. If a woman with an underactive thyroid succeeds in becoming pregnant, she must continue to take the appropriate doses of supplemental thyroid hormone. Otherwise, her fetus may be adversely affected.

The most important point about the treatment of hypothyroidism is that treatment should be determined by how the patient feels, rather than by the levels of thyroid hormone in her blood. Even if the patient's blood levels become normal, if her symptoms improve marginallly, she may require higher doses of thyroid medication. In fact, the treatment of hypothyroidism is similar to cooking: a great chef does not merely follow a recipe but modifies it according to the unique ingredients available on a particular day. So too should the treatment of hypothyroidism be modified according to a patient's unique symptoms. It is also critical to remember that when the thyroid is underactive, it remains so for life. Treatment must never be stopped and will probably need to be adjusted periodically, depending on how the patient feels.

Hyperthyroidism (overactive thyroid) is a much more rare condition. It can result in a medical emergency and must be treated promptly, usually by drinking a radioactive iodine cocktail that destroys the over-functioning thyroid tissue. Most often, the patient then becomes hypothyroid and will require some degree of thyroid hormone replacement. The usual symptoms of hyperthyroidism are very heavy menstrual periods, weight loss, unusual nervousness, insomnia, heart palpitations and profuse sweating.

OVULATION TESTS

Currently, the best way to assess accurately whether ovulation is taking place is via vaginal ultrasound. The more traditional methods of detecting and/or predicting ovulation, i.e., measurement of a woman's basal body temperature (BBT) or urine testing for LH, can be time-consuming, may provide inconsistent results and are generally unreliable. In fact, one study has indicated that home ovulation kits are inaccurate about 20% of the time.

By examining a patient via sonogram at various times during her menstrual cycle, the doctor can determine whether or not she is producing follicles (each of which presumably contains an egg) and whether they are able to be released from the ovaries. For example, if a woman has a 30-day cycle, a sonogram performed on day 14 or 15 should show a mature, 20-mm follicle in the ovary. A follow-up sonogram performed 48 hours later should show that the follicle has burst and that the egg has been released. The doctor can also use a sonogram to see whether the woman's endometrium (uterine lining) is developing normally over the course of her menstrual cycle.

HYSTEROSALPINGOGRAM (HSG)

Since blocked Fallopian tubes are responsible for preventing pregnancy in up to 30% of infertile couples, the next step in the workup would probably be a hysterosalpingogram (HSG), a special kind of x-ray that is 85-90% accurate in diagnosing tubal blockages. An HSG can also diagnose a hydrosalpinx (fluid in the tubes).

To perform an HSG, a doctor injects a dye through the woman's cervix and into her uterus and Fallopian tubes. A series of x-ray pictures of the pelvic region are taken as the dye is being injected. If a woman's tubes are open, the x-rays will show the dye flowing freely out of the ends and into her abdominal cavity, where it will be absorbed. If the dye cannot flow freely, the tube is blocked.

An HSG may cause discomfort. The patient will probably feel a sense of pressure as the dye is injected. The dye injection will also cause cramping and lower abdominal pain. This generally subsides shortly after the procedure has been completed. Also, over-the-counter pain relievers such as Advil™ or other non-steroidal anti-inflammatory drugs taken one to two hours before the procedure can help prevent most of the discomfort.

Women with iodine (shellfish) allergies will be allergic to the dye used in an HSG. For such patients, the doctor might utilize ultrasound, injecting the tubes with saline (salt water) instead of the dye to visually check whether the Fallopian tubes are open.

What the X-Ray May Not Show

Even if an HSG shows that the patient's tubes appear to be open, they may still not function normally. There is no test—not even the insertion of a small telescope (falloposcope) into the tubes—that can show how well the tubes perform. Therefore, it is important not to rule out the possibility of tubal damage as a cause of a woman's infertility despite the presence of a normal HSG.

A condition called a hydrosalpinx is present when an HSG shows that fluid has accumulated in the Fallopian tube. The blockage usually occurs at the far, fimbriated end of the Fallopian tube, which becomes sealed as a result of scar tissue formation. Most often, a hydrosalpinx results from a prior chlamydial or other bacterial infection, and the patient may have a positive anti-chlamydial antibody blood test. The fluid that accumulates in the tube contains no active bacteria or viruses, but it does contain many protein substances. The presence of a hydrosalpinx indicates that the tubal lining, which is vital to the fertilization process, is irrevocably damaged.

There is anecdotal evidence that some women will conceive after an HSG if oil-based (rather than water-based) dye solution is used. Some theories suggest that the pressure of the thick solution may mechanically "flush out" the tubes. We believe that the oil-based dye attracts the scavenger cells in a woman's immune system. This temporarily diverts them from being attracted to and attacking the sperm and egg, thereby allowing conception to take place in some patients. Pregnancies that occur after an HSG are probably coincidental and are not actually a result of the procedure. Therefore, patients should not undergo an HSG in order to conceive. Also, it is important to be aware that there is a fair amount of x-ray exposure during an HSG, especially when fluoroscopy (the x-ray is seen on a screen in real time during the procedure) is used.

HYDROSONOGRAM

A hydrosonogram is a vaginal ultrasound in which saline (salt water) is introduced into the uterine cavity. If the Fallopian tubes are open, the fluid will be seen to have flowed out of the tubes and into the pelvis. If there is a blockage, no fluid will be seen passing into the pelvic cavity. Many fertility specialists now recommend a hydrosonogram as the preliminary test of choice to evaluate tubal patency and the uterine cavity. Several valid reasons support this recommendation. First, a hydrosonogram is usually less painful than an HSG. Also, there are virtually no allergic reactions associated with saline. Finally, with a hydrosonogram, a patient is not exposed to x-rays, while an HSG requires a considerable amount of x-ray exposure. Although an HSG can usually better pinpoint the location of tubal blockages than a hydrosonogram, this is less critical, as surgical removal of such blockages (tubalplasty) is not very effective and is rarely performed in contemporary medical practice.

POST-COITAL TEST: OFTEN IGNORED, BUT OF DEFINITE SIGNIFICANCE

A post-coital test (PCT) provides important information as to the amount of a male's sperm as well as its ability to reach and survive in a female's cervical mucus at the entrance of the uterus. Seeing sperm swimming in the cervical mucus is like having a runner on first base: if there is no runner on first base, it is not possible to score! So a good PCT indicates that pregnancy is a possibility, whereas a poor one is an indication that there may be a male problem or that the female's mucus is a barrier to conception.

For the PCT, a couple is instructed to have intercourse around the time of ovulation, when the mucus is most copious. The woman is then asked to visit the doctor's office 12 to 24 hours afterward, so that a sample of her mucus can be observed under a microscope. When the test is performed too long before ovulation or one day after, the cervical mucus will be too scant or too thick to provide an accurate result. Obviously, the test isn't painful and can easily evaluate the male factor, especially if a man is reticent about providing a sperm sample for a formal semen analysis.

By examining and counting the sperm in the sample, a physician can determine whether the male's sperm can survive in his partner's cervical mucus and whether they are strong enough to make it through the vagina and cervical canal to enter the uterus and tubes. If the couple has excellent results on the PCT, intrauterine insemination (IUI) will probably not help in the process of conception. Yet the mere presence of many sperm at the entrance of the womb is no guarantee that they have been able to swim to the site where fertilization occurs. I believe that the PCT is a simple, yet critical test; like any other diagnostic test, however, it is not infallible. I have actually seen pregnancies occurring in cycles in which the PCT result was poor.

THE SUCCESS-ORIENTED WORKUP FOR HIM

The recent development of Intracytoplasmic Sperm Injection (ICSI), a procedure in which a single sperm is injected directly into the egg to cause fertilization, has revolutionized the diagnosis and treatment of male infertility and eliminated the need for most of the traditional fertility tests and procedures for men. With the success-oriented approach, only a few tests remain necessary for the male.

PATIENT HISTORY

A male's health and reproductive history can help the doctor determine whether or not the couple should begin with the earlier steps in *The Pregnancy Prescription* or proceed directly to IVF, most often using Intracyoplasmic Sperm Injection (ICSI—discussed in Chapter 9).

The most important element of a male's history is whether he has created a pregnancy—either naturally or via IVF—during the past ten years. If so, this strongly implies that his sperm, no matter what the count, should be biologically capable of fertilizing an egg. This may not be true of a man who has had a vasectomy reversal in the intervening years since the pregnancy, as in some cases post-vasectomy sperm may not be able to achieve fertilization normally.

Another signal that there may be a problem with the sperm supply is a history of undescended testes, or diseases such as mumps, epididymitis (infection of the epididymis) or prostatitis (infection of the prostate gland). Past exposure to such harmful substances as lead, cigarette smoke, marijuana or excessive alcohol are said to adversely affect sperm quality in some men, but there are no observable ill effects in many others.

SEMEN ANALYSIS

Traditionally, semen analysis has been the key diagnostic exam for men. For this test, the male is asked to ejaculate into a sterile container—usually while he is in the doctor's office or lab. Men who feel too inhibited to bring themselves to ejaculate in such a foreign environment should be permitted to produce the specimen at home, as long as it is brought to the doctor's office in a specified time period, keeping the sample at room temperature and following all other instructions. Within three hours of producing the specimen, a computerized semen analysis can provide information as to the quantity of living, moving sperm, motility (movement), velocity (speed) and morphology (shape). A sperm specimen does not even begin to deteriorate for at least three hours from the time of collection, as long as it is not exposed to very cold temperatures. You do not have to run through any red lights in order to get the specimen to the lab before all the sperm die!!

Unfortunately, semen analysis has proven disappointing in differentiating between which men can produce a pregnancy and which cannot, since many men with poor-quality sperm succeed in fathering children naturally. In reality, no particular parameter in the sperm count can provide an accurate indication of a male's fertility—with the possible exception of velocity, which we have found to be an accurate predictor of the sperm's potential ability to fertilize an egg. If, after processing and incubation, a male's sperm are found to swim slower than 60 microns per second, it has been our experience that the sperm will be unable to fertilize an egg on their own and the embryologist will need to perform ICSI to achieve fertilization for that couple.

THE ULTIMATE FERTILITY TEST: *IN VITRO* FERTILIZATION

As a diagnostic test, IVF provides the doctor with the most accurate indication of where the reproductive process is going awry. For example, if a couple fails to conceive through intercourse or intrauterine insemination and the woman has one or more diagnosed fertility problems (e.g., a single blocked tube, endometriosis), it would be logical to assume that one of these problems has been preventing her from conceiving. But if the same woman's eggs fail to fertilize during a diagnostic IVF cycle, it is clear that those problems were not the only ones keeping her from becoming pregnant, but were "red herrings." The underlying problem preventing fertilization and conception might have gone undetected had it not been for the diagnostic ability of IVF.

SUCCESS-ORIENTED TREATMENT DECISIONS

Here are a few examples of how a success-oriented physician might use the information provided by these tests to determine the best course of treatment for an infertile couple.

Blocked Fallopian Tubes

If an HSG indicated that one or both of the woman's Fallopian tubes were blocked, the doctor would probably decide to bypass the tubes altogether and proceed directly to IVF. Theoretically, surgery could be performed to remove the blockages. However, undetectable and untreatable damage could remain to prevent the couple from conceiving naturally. Therefore, the doctor would probably elect not to perform a laparoscopy or any other surgical procedure to attempt to open the tubes, instead bypassing them altogether.

Highly Positive Anti-Chlamydia Antibody Tests/Normal HSG

If an HSG showed the woman's tubes to be open, but she was still unable to conceive despite all other factors being normal except for high levels of anti-Chlamydia antibodies, the doctor could reasonably assume that the cellular linings of her Fallopian tubes had been damaged—since the blood tests for anti-chlamydia antibodies were strongly positive, revealing a prior, nonsymptomatic Chlamydia infection. In this case, the doctor would probably elect to bypass the Fallopian tubes, which were the most likely source of the patient's inability to conceive, and proceed directly to IVF.

Consistently High FSH Levels

If a woman's day 2 to 3 FSH level were consistently as high as 20-25 mlU/mL (or even 15 mlU/mL), her prognosis for pregnancy with her own eggs would be considered poor. The doctor might counsel the couple to consider using donor eggs if they still wanted to try for a pregnancy.

Failure to Ovulate

If a series of sonograms showed that a woman was unable to develop and/or release eggs on her own, the doctor would obviously elect to begin treatment with oral fertility drugs to help her ovulate. The stimulation of ovulation would often be combined with intrauterine insemination to increase the chances of her partner's sperm meeting up with an egg. If the couple failed to conceive after three to four cycles, the doctor might advise proceeding directly to a diagnostic IVF cycle, since 85% of all conceptions occur within the first three treatment cycles.

Poor Post-Coital Test

If the results of the PCT were poor, the couple would be advised to try intrauterine insemination to bypass the cervical mucus—usually combining IUI with fertility drugs to increase the chances of conception. If three to four cycles of this treatment failed to produce a pregnancy, the doctor would advise the couple to proceed to a diagnostic/therapeutic IVF cycle.

Good Post-Coital Test/Failure To Conceive

If a patient who ovulates regularly has been unable to conceive and has excellent PCT results, insemination will not increase her chances of becoming pregnant. The presence of an excellent post-coital test indicates that the sperm are capable of arriving in the proximity of the egg. It does not indicate whether or not the sperm are actually capable of fertilizing the oocyte. These patients should proceed directly to IVF, since their problem is most likely one of fertilization failure or embryo quality.

Low Sperm Velocity/No Conception With Fertility Drugs and Insemination

The doctor would assume that the sperm is unable to

fertilize the egg and would counsel the couple to proceed directly to IVF with ICSI.

An IVF Cycle with No Fertilization

During a standard IVF cycle, if a couple with normal-looking eggs and sperm did not achieve fertilization during the first 24 hours after retrieval, the embryologist might attempt to inject the sperm directly into the eggs (ICSI) on the second day of the cycle. If this succeeded in causing fertilization, the cycle could be salvaged, although pregnancy rates are much lower with ICSI performed on the day after egg retrieval. In this case, it would be difficult to determine whether the initial fertilization failure was due to a problem with the egg or the sperm. If fertilization failed to occur after the second-day ICSI, during the couple's next IVF cycle the couple might elect to fertilize 50% of the eggs with the partner's sperm via ICSI and leave the remaining eggs to be fertilized in the normal manner, using donor sperm. The results would be interpreted as follows:

FERTILIZATION OUTCOME		
DONOR SPERM	**PARTNER'S SPERM/ ICSI**	**IMPLICATION**
No	No	Egg problem: consider donor eggs
Yes	Yes	Partner's sperm had egg-binding problem
Yes	No	Probable genetic problem with partner's sperm

DIAGNOSTIC TESTS THAT HAVE BEEN ELIMINATED FROM THE STREAMLINED WORKUP

Physical Examination

Rarely, if ever, will a significant abnormality affecting reproduction be detected during a physical exam. If a woman has undergone a normal gynecological exam and pap smear within the previous 12 months, a pelvic sonogram is the only physical examination she needs.

Cultures

It has been standard for doctors to take cervical cultures to check for infection by relevant organisms such as chlamydia. But the presence of infection with any organism other than chlamydia or gonorrhea has never been proven to cause infertility. Therefore, an extensive bacteriologic evaluation of a couple, plus prolonged, "heavy duty" antibiotic therapy, is not indicated—and may even be dangerous. Besides, a negative culture indicates only that the patient is suffering no current infection. A previous infection with chlamydia or gonorrhea could have affected her ability to conceive by damaging the Fallopian tubes. And since these organisms may not cause noticeable symptoms (or if there were symptoms, the patient may have attributed them to another cause), simply asking the woman if she has ever had a pelvic infection won't always provide accurate information. The only way to accurately assess whether or not the patient has experienced a previous pelvic infection that may have affected her fertility is via a blood test for the anti-chlamydia antibody.

Inhibin B/ Anti-Mullerian Hormone (AMH)

Measurment of these hormones in a woman's blood may offer some predictive insight into the number of eggs that she will produce with ovarian stimulation. Nevertheless, in my opinion, these tests are redundant and quite unnecessary, because the measurement of ovarian reserve sonographically will accurately predict the number of egg follicles that a woman will produce with maximal ovarian stimulation. In addition, constantly high levels of FSH also indicate that few or no eggs will be produced. Lastly, these tests are not routinely performed by most clinical laboratories, nor are they covered by most medical insurances.

Ovulation Tests

In the past, a physician may have tried to assess whether a fertility patient was ovulating by asking her to keep monthly charts of her basal (first-thing-in-the-morning) body temperature (BBT) to determine whether it showed the mid-cycle rise that normally follows ovulation. Or the doctor may have asked her to perform a series of at-home ovulation tests or measured the level of progesterone in her blood during the latter part of her cycle, again to determine whether it showed the elevation that typically follows ovulation. Unfortunately, none of these tests are precise. The BBT, in particular, is time consuming and can document ovulation only after it has occurred. Today we know that the most effective and efficient way to document ovulation is to actually view egg follicle development directly via a vaginal sonogram. However, as mentioned earlier, a BBT that is consistently lower than 97.5 F in the days prior to ovulation strongly suggests an underactive thyroid gland. Not infrequently, a new patient who brings in months of temperature charts is surprised to learn how useful they are in helping to diagnose her previously undetected hypothyroidism!

Endometrial Biopsy

Endometrial biopsy (examination of the lining of the uterus) has traditionally been performed as a means of diagnosing luteal phase defects (insufficient progesterone production during the second half of the menstrual cycle) and evaluating the ability of the patient's uterine lining to support an implanted embryo.

Many physicians have now abandoned the endometrial biopsy, since vaginal ultrasound has provided them with a more sophisticated and less invasive means of evaluating the growth patterns of the patient's endometrium.

Laparoscopy

Diagnostic laparoscopy (a surgical procedure that allows the doctor to actually look inside the woman's abdominal cavity to view her pelvic organs) was once a standard component of any infertility evaluation. Laparoscopy is performed while the patient is under general anesthesia. The doctor makes several small incisions in the woman's abdomen and inflates the cavity with a small amount of carbon dioxide gas to make her organs more easily visible. A small camera, attached to a telescope, is inserted through one of the incisions. This allows the doctor to view the woman's internal anatomy on a nearby video screen. The other incisions provide access for the doctor's instruments and surgical tools.

Physicians would generally perform a laparoscopy to see if there were any signs of scar tissue or endometriosis in the woman's pelvic area, in addition to confirming tubal blockages that had been diagnosed via an HSG. If any adhesions or signs of endometriosis were found, they could be resolved during this diagnostic procedure. If the woman failed to conceive after the laparoscopy, a second might be performed to see if the blockages or adhesions had re-occurred. Whether this type of surgery is justified as a diagnostic and treatment tool for infertility has never been proven. For one thing, an estimated 95% of laparoscopies performed for diagnostic purposes reveal nothing to be wrong. Second, even if a problem, such as endometriosis, is detected, there is no proof that correcting it will increase a patient's chances of conceiving. Although endometriosis seems to be associated with fertility problems, it has never been established as a cause of infertility. Women who are diagnosed with endometriosis and treated with fertility drugs and insemination have been shown to become pregnant just as often as those treated with surgery and drugs. In fact, no medical or surgical treatment of endometriosis has been shown substantially to increase fertility rates. Since laparoscopy is a surgical procedure that adds little to helping a couple conceive, I believe that its risks outweigh its benefits. Therefore, I advise patients to avoid undergoing laparoscopy as a part of their fertility evaluation.

Anti-Sperm Antibody Tests

There has been no definitive evidence that the presence of anti-sperm antibodies (detected via blood tests or when they are found coating the heads of the spermatozoa) causes infertility or that the success rates of either intrauterine insemination or IVF are lower in women with anti-sperm antibodies. In fact, 15% of couples that have had successful pregnancies have tested positive for anti-sperm antibodies.

Hamster Egg Penetration Test

A "high-tech" test of male fertility has been the Hamster Egg Penetration Test. This test requires hamster eggs to be stripped of their outer shells (zona pellucida) and exposed to a human sperm sample. The number of sperm that penetrate the hamster egg has been considered a measure of the male's fertility.

Clinical experience has shown the hamster test to be unreliable. For one thing, in humans, sperm need to bind onto and penetrate the zona pellucida. This ability can't be tested in the hamster test since hamster eggs need to be stripped of their shells in order for human sperm to gain entry. Furthermore, experience has shown that a significant percentage of men who are unable to fertilize hamster eggs can fertilize their partners' eggs *in vitro*, either with or without ICSI.

Sperm DNA Tests

Tests for the structural integrity of sperm DNA have been developed in order to identify men who may be infertile despite having a normal semen analysis. In other words, although a man's sperm cells appear to be normal in all respects when examined under a microscope, a relatively high proportion of the spermatozoa could contain abnormal DNA. Theoretically, when a sperm cell bearing abnormal DNA fertilizes an egg, the resulting embryo must be genetically imperfect. This type of test is of potential scientific interest; it is of questionable clinical value for several reasons. The most compelling one is that pregnancies are achieved by the partners of men who are identified by the test to have a high proportion of sperm with abnormal DNA. Second, even if a man has a high proportion of abnormal DNA sperm cells, there is no known medical therapy for this supposed abnormality. Why, then, test for a condition that has no remedy? Since no one actually has 100% abnormal DNA in each and every sperm cell that he has—or ever will—produce, an abnormal result does not mean that he will never father his own biological child. At most, I believe, sperm testing of this sort may identify individuals who may take longer to impregnate their partners. This test seems to me to be interesting as a research tool, but it has no practical clinical value.

THE MINIMALIST APPROACH TO THE EVALUATION AND TREATMENT OF INFERTILITY

A different approach to infertility treatment—the minimalist approach—is the most streamlined method of overcoming infertility. The minimalist approach to the infertile couple evolved in Japan, where it is widely used. This approach is Zen-like, since it advocates simplicity and gentleness in both diagnosis and treatment. There are only four basic tests used in the minimalist approach to determine the starting point for infertility treatment: a post-coital test, an HSG or Hydrosonogram, an anti-chlamydial antibody level to evaluate the status of the Fallopian tubes and a pelvic sonogram to document ovulation and ovarian reserve. A semen analysis is performed only if the post-coital test is abnormal to determine whether there is a mild or serious deficiency in the sperm count or motility. Similar to the success-oriented approach, laparoscopy is considered unnecessary.

The minimalist approach was created by Dr. Osamu Kato—the founder of a large fertility clinic in Tokyo. It is mainly based on theories he has adopted from his vast clinical experience and the invaluable store of knowledge that comes from treating a large number of infertile couples. Some physicians may be critical of his approach because it is not based entirely on scientific research. However, medicine is both an art and a science. I believe that the art of medicine—an intuitive ability, combined with years of clinical experience—is just as important to the proper treatment of patients as is the purely scientific part of medical practice.

The minimalist approach differs philosophically in certain ways from both the success-oriented and the traditionalist approaches to infertility, especially with regard to the cause and treatment of unexplained infertility. The major difference, according to Dr. Kato, is that unexplained infertility is caused by a failure of egg pick-up because of a functional defect of the Fallopian tubes. Therefore, he believes, the failure of conception is due to the inability of the sperm and egg to meet, hence fertilization cannot occur. This is in sharp conflict with the mainstream school of thought, which posits that failure of conception is mainly due to genetic abnormalities of the fertilized eggs that preclude them from developing into healthy babies. I believe that perhaps both theories contain elements of truth. In certain couples, the inability of the Fallopian tubes to pick up eggs properly could be the problem, whereas other cases of unexplained infertility could be caused by embryonic genetic abnormalities resulting from oocyte quality issues. Actually, neither theory can be scientifically proven or disproven. In the final analysis, it really doesn't matter why you can't conceive, just as long as there are treatments available that will help you have a baby! The bottom line is that both the minimalist and the success-oriented physicians agree that IVF is the best way to confront the problem of unexplained infertility. If a woman's problem is due to a fertilization failure resulting from faulty egg pick-up, using IVF, her eggs will fertilize, her embryos will appear healthy and pregnancy should occur within two or three treatment cycles. If the underlying cause of a patient's unexplained infertility is embryonic genetic abnormalities, IVF will show poor embryo growth or quality. If conception does not occur even when the embryos appear healthy in terms of growth and microscopic structure, embryonic genetic analysis can be performed with Preimplantation Genetic Diagnosis (PGD—discussed in Chapter 12). In these cases, only the genetically normal (to the extent that genetically normal embryos can be identified) will be transferred.

SUMMARY

Since success-oriented physicians believe that most of the problems that cause infertility are impossible to diagnose and treat, the success-oriented workup will usually consist of only a few basic, non-invasive tests to rule out obvious causes of infertility. If you are following the minimalist approach, the workup will be even slightly more abbreviated. These workups will help a doctor determine which form of treatment is the best starting point for you and your partner. Both success-oriented physicians as well as those who are proponents of the minimalist approach believe in using IVF early on as both a diagnostic and treatment tool. This knowledge should help save you significant time, pain, and expense in resolving your infertility problems.

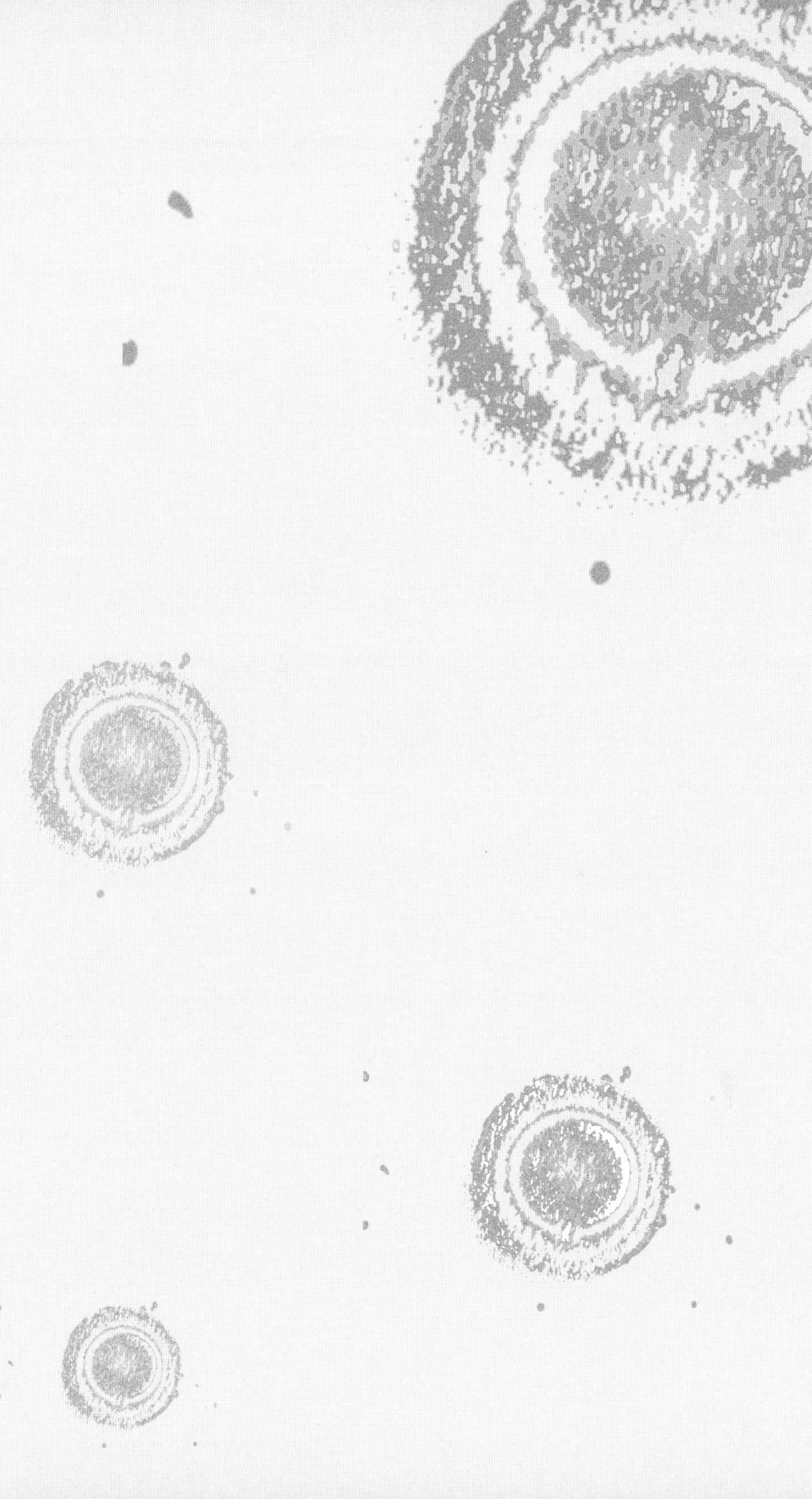

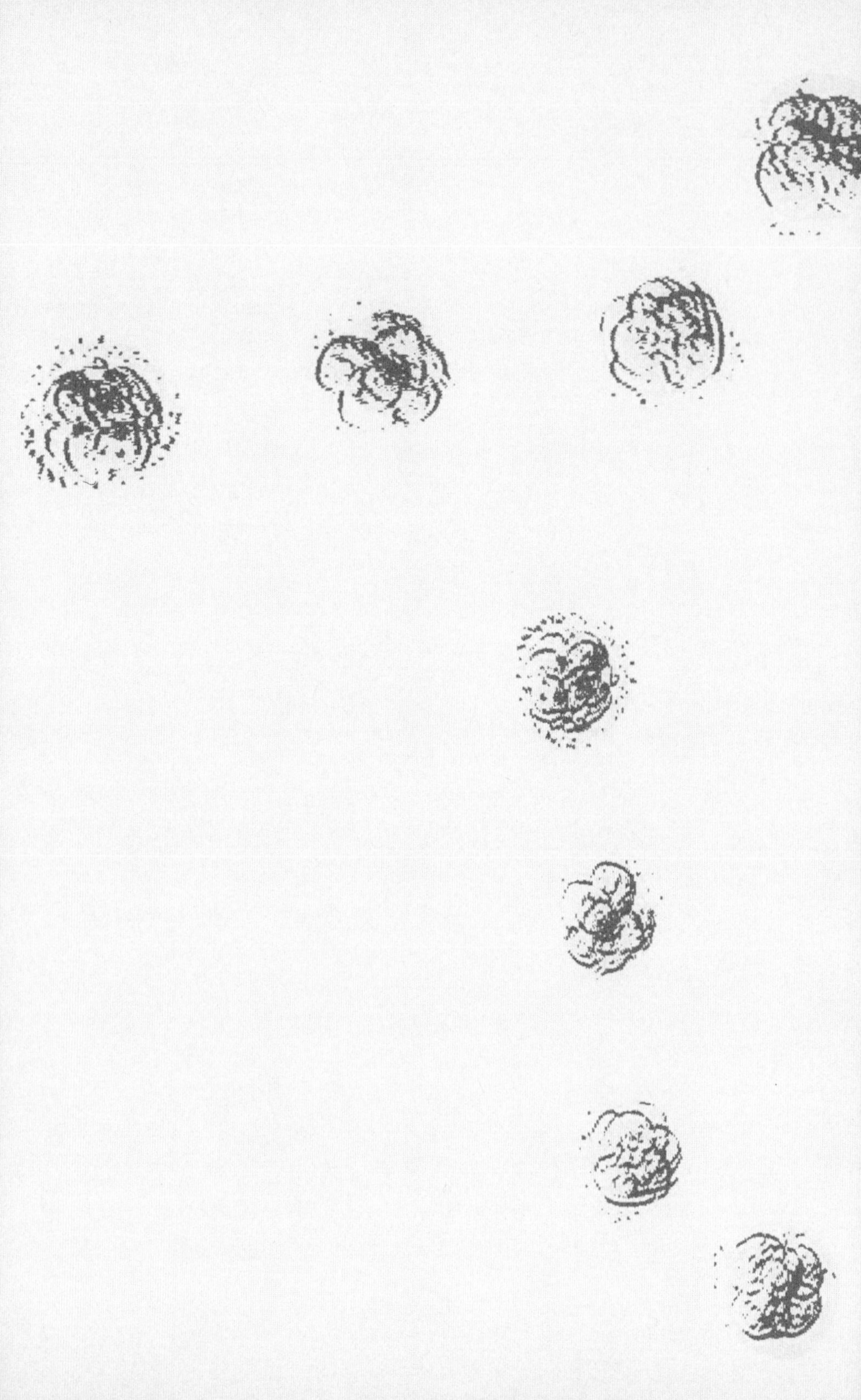

CHAPTER 5

STEP 1

The Treatment of Infertility Oral Fertility Drugs and Intrauterine Insemination (IUI)

The next step in the quest for pregnancy is a combination treatment of the oral fertility drug, Clomiphene Citrate (brand names: Clomid, Serophene), and Intrauterine Insemination (IUI). Although either treatment alone might help some couples, conception is more likely if the fertility drug and insemination are combined.

This step may be a good starting point for you and your partner if the results of your streamlined workup suggest any of the following:

FOR HER

- Failure to ovulate, infrequent ovulatory cycles, irregular periods
- Medical history suggests mild endometriosis
- Open Fallopian tubes

FOR HIM

- A slightly low sperm count (10-20 million)
- Decreased sperm velocity (speed of <30 microns per second) prior to processing
- An increased number of sperm with abnormal morphology (shape)
- Poor post-coital test

FOR BOTH

- Unexplained infertility of more than one-year duration

ORAL FERTILITY DRUGS

Clomiphene Citrate

Clomiphene Citrate (Clomid, Serophene) is an oral fertility drug that initiates a process called Controlled Ovarian Hyperstimulation (COH), or superovulation, in women with normal ovulation. In COH with clomiphene citrate, the drug stimulates the hypothalamus—the control system in the brain—to produce GNRF (Gonadotropin Releasing Factor) that, in turn, causes the pituitary gland to produce additional FSH and LH. These hormones stimulate the ovary to produce greater numbers of oocytes. In this way, clomiphene citrate encourages conception by helping the woman to produce additional "targets" for her partner's sperm.

How It Evolved

Clomiphene Citrate was the first fertility drug to become available in the US. Ironically, clomiphene was first tested for use as a birth control pill in the 1960s. When women taking the drug were found to have an exceptionally high rate of conception, researchers decided that the best use of clomiphene would be as a means of enhancing, rather than preventing, pregnancy. Believe it or not, this fertility drug has been in use for 50 years!

Clomiphene was used to treat infertile women in whom the pituitary gland and/or hypothalamus were unable to stimulate the production of FSH and LH, rendering it impossible for them to either ovulate or menstruate. Eventually, doctors started prescribing clomiphene to help increase the number of follicles produced by women who did ovulate normally, in order to increase their chances for conception.

Clomiphene Citrate as Treatment

Today, the normally prescribed dosage of clomiphene is 100 mg (two 50-mg tablets) per day for five to seven days, beginning on day 2 or 3 of the woman's menstrual cycle. In most cases, doses higher than 100 to 150 mg per day will not increase the number of follicles. Women who weigh more than 200 lbs may need more than the standard dosage, and very thin women may require only 50 mg per day.

Clomiphene Citrate for Diagnostic Testing

Clomiphene can also be used to predict a woman's potential to become pregnant. For this purpose, she would take two clomiphene tablets per day, starting on day 2 to 3 of her menstrual cycle, after which her ovaries would be examined via vaginal ultrasound. If the sonogram showed that she was able to produce as many as three to six mature egg follicles, it would mean that she was very responsive to the drug and would probably have a good chance of becoming pregnant. If she were to produce only one follicle, it would indicate that her ability to produce eggs was possibly compromised and her chances for pregnancy could be reduced, regardless of her chronological age.

Another test, the "clomiphene challenge test," calls for the woman to take two clomiphene tablets on days 5 to 9 of her cycle and then have her FSH level tested on day 10. If the blood test showed her FSH level to be 26 or greater (the normal response would be ≤15), her potential for becoming pregnant would be minimal.

Women who fare poorly on either of these tests will

probably not respond well to even the more potent forms of ovarian stimulation, the gonadotropins, and may need to consider other options for expanding their families.

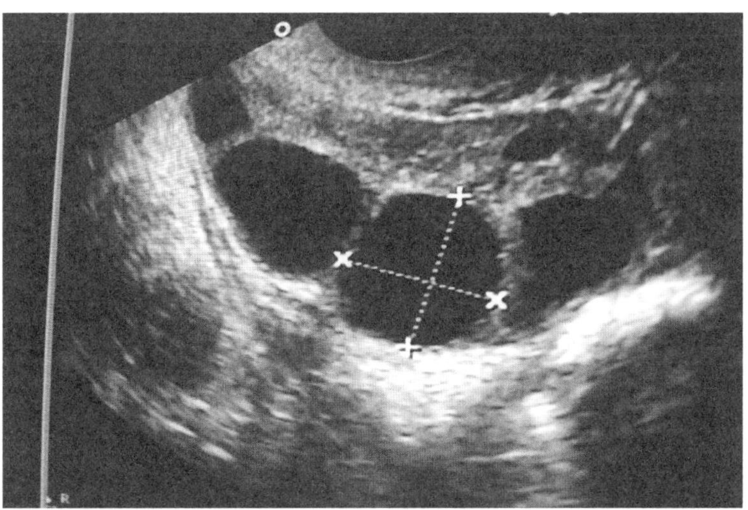

Fig. 1. ***Three egg follicles stimulated by Clomid 100mg/ day for five days.***

Pros and Cons of Clomiphene Citrate

Clomiphene is a relatively inexpensive drug with limited side effects. The drug usually avoids over-stimulating (hyperstimulating) the ovaries, thus making it an extremely safe treatment option. **<u>No causal link has ever been proven between fertility drugs and ovarian or breast cancer</u>.** However, one study did note a slightly higher incidence of ovarian cancer in women who took clomiphene citrate for more than 12 months. Since clomiphene, if it will work, will produce a pregnancy in three to four cycles, our recommendation is that women not use the drug for more than four months.

On the days clomiphene is taken, patients may experience hot flushes, mood swings, headaches, or slight visual disturbances. There is a small risk that clomiphene will have a drying effect on the cervical and endometrial mucus or cause the uterine lining to thin to the extent that it could prevent an embryo from implanting. These problems can be diagnosed via a post-coital test and/or ultrasound at the time of insemination. If the cervical mucus appears to have been adversely affected by clomiphene, it is possible that the mucus lining the uterus and Fallopian tubes have also been negatively affected. These are completely reversed during subsequent "non-clomiphene" cycles. Women experiencing such negative effects should discontinue treatment and use other fertility drugs in subsequent cycles.

Other Options

In some patients, the problems that may be associated with clomiphene can be avoided by using similar drugs.

Letrozole (Femara®) is currently the most popular alternative to clomiphene. Letrozole does not dry the cervical mucus or adversely affect the endometrial lining. The usual dose is 5.0 mg daily for five to seven days, beginning on day 2 or 3 of the menstrual cycle. Some patients with polycystic ovaries may be treated with letrozole on a daily basis until a mature follicle develops. In some patients, this may take three to four weeks. Unlike treatment with clomiphene, HCG must be given when the patient's follicle reaches 20 mm in size since an LH surge does not occur naturally with the use of letrozole. Consequently, a patient will not release a mature egg without some form of HCG being injected.

This protocol is an acceptable choice for IUI, but is not potent enough for ovarian stimulation for IVF.

Tamoxifen citrate (Nolvadex™), best known as an anti-breast cancer drug, works in much the same way as does clomiphene, but without causing the drying effect in the mucus. This drug, in combination with injectable fertility drugs (gonadotropins), is the drug of choice for IVF in women who have had breast cancer. Tamoxifen is available in 10-mg tablets, and the usual dosage is 30-40 mg for five days, starting on day 2 or 3 of the menstrual cycle.

Pharmacists are often confused when tamoxifen is substituted for clomid and used for fertility treatment. However, although it is not recognized as an ovulation-inducing agent by the FDA, tamoxifen has been found to work well for this purpose and is less expensive than clomiphene.

INTRAUTERINE INSEMINATION (IUI)

In Intrauterine Insemination (IUI), processed semen is placed into the woman's uterus around the time that she ovulates. IUI helps to increase the chances for conception in two ways. First, pre-insemination processing helps to increase the concentration and velocity (speed) of the sperm while weeding out potential "underachievers." Then the insemination process itself makes it possible for the processed sperm to be deposited much closer to the oocyte than normal intercourse would permit, bypassing any potential problems in the vagina and/or cervix.

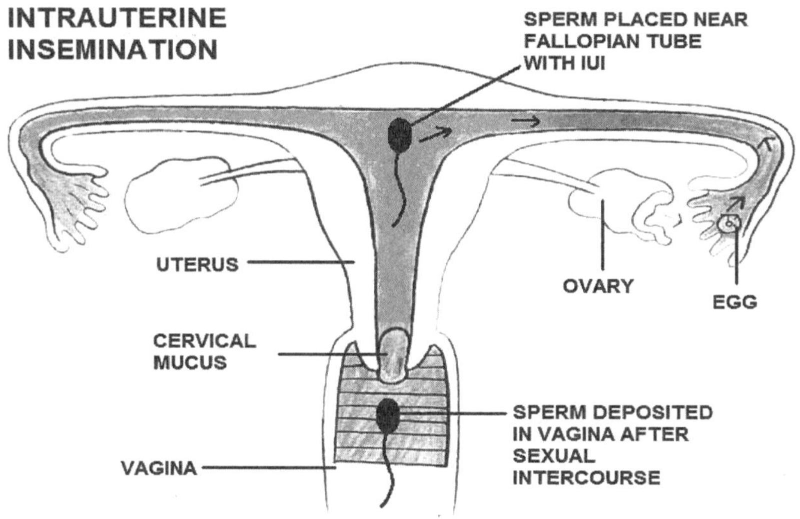

Fig. 2. ***Intrauterine insemination puts the sperm in closer proximity to the egg.***

How IUI Evolved

Insemination is not a new treatment for infertility. The first recorded inseminations were performed in the 1790s, when the male's ejaculate was mechanically deposited into a woman's vagina. From that time until the 1950s, all inseminations were carried out intravaginally, with the same "turkey baster" technique. From the 1950s through the 1970s, intravaginal insemination was replaced by intracervical insemination, in which an unprocessed ejaculate was placed into the woman's cervix so that it could mix directly with her cervical mucus. In the early 1980s, physicians discovered that adding tissue culture media (a nutrient broth used to grow and maintain living cells in a laboratory setting) to the semen increased the speed with which the sperm could swim. This was found to be a way for men with low sperm counts or poor motility to increase their chances for impregnating their partners. To further enhance the odds for conception, doctors began inserting the processed sperm into the woman's uterus, bypassing the vagina and cervix completely.

Producing the Specimen

Around the time that the woman is ovulating, the male produces a sperm specimen by ejaculating into a small, sterile container. This can be done either at the doctor's office or at home. Since normal latex condoms will kill sperm, the sample should be produced through masturbation rather than via intercourse with a condom. The physician can provide special non-latex condoms to men with religious or personal aversions to masturbation, but this method is likely to result in a good portion of the specimen being lost.

If the specimen is produced at home, it is important to keep it at room temperature until it reaches the lab, avoiding any extremes of hot or cold. In winter, one trick for keeping the sample warm is for the woman to place the closed container inside her bra, enabling her natural body heat to protect it.

The specimen should arrive at the doctor's office within three hours after it has been produced. After that time it may begin to deteriorate, but it is important to remember that each and every sperm will not self-destruct at exactly 180 minutes after ejaculation. Even after deterioration has begun, some "resurrection" will occur during the processing and incubation that is part of the standard sperm processing procedure.

Processing the Semen

Once the sperm specimen arrives at the office, it can be processed through a number of techniques. The specific processing technique used is not critical as long as the culture medium is fresh and its acid/base balance (pH) is appropriately adjusted, since any deviation will kill the sperm. The sperm specimen is mixed with culture medium and is spun in a centrifuge to separate the sperm from the seminal fluid in which it was ejaculated. The seminal plasma and the initial medium is removed and replaced with fresh culture medium. The specimen is then placed in an incubator so that the best "swimmers" are concentrated in the fresh medium. As a result of the processing procedure, a highly concentrated population of the most active sperm is made available for insemination directly into the top of the partner's uterus. If a small amount of seminal plasma remains in the processed sperm specimen, a woman may experience an inflammatory reaction that could cause temporary cramping, diarrhea or even fever after the insemination (a rare occurrence). These reactions result from substances called prostaglandins and will usually resolve spontaneously in one to two hours. Ibuprophen (Motrin) will help these distressing but harmless symptoms disappear rapidly. This type of reaction is quite different from an infection caused by the transfer of bacteria into the uterus. Bacteria and other cellular elements are removed during the washing process. As an additional safeguard to prevent the possibility of infection, antibiotics are added to the processing medium to eliminate any remaining bacteria.

The Procedure

After the sperm processing is completed, which takes between 45 minutes and 2 hours, the insemination is relatively easy. The woman lies on an examining table in the usual position for a gynecological exam and a speculum is inserted into her vagina so that the doctor can access her cervix. The doctor draws the sperm specimen up into soft plastic tubing with a syringe and then passes the tubing through the cervical opening. The woman may experience one slight cramp as the catheter passes through the cervix and another when the catheter reaches the top of her uterus. In many instances, doctors use abdominal ultrasound to help guide its placement. Once the catheter is in place, approximately 1 to 2 cc. of processed sperm is released into the uterus. The sperm specimen often reaches the midpoint of the Fallopian tube when it is delivered into the upper segment of the uterine cavity. IUI gives the sperm a great "head start" in its quest to reach the egg.

Although it rarely happens, IUI may cause an infection in the woman's uterus or Fallopian tubes. If she experiences chills, low abdominal pain or an oral temperature greater than 101°F within 12 to 24 hours of the insemination, she should contact her doctor. Antibiotics administered on a timely basis can prevent permanent damage from occurring.

Exact Timing Is Not Necessary

IUI needs to take place when the woman is most likely to be ovulating, but there is no need for the couple to time the insemination for the exact moment the egg is "dropped." There is actually a wide time frame during which fertilization can take place.

Most women will begin using a home urine test for predicting ovulation on day 10 of their cycle. (Women with shorter cycles lasting 25-26 days should start on day 7.) When the results of the test are positive (meaning the LH surge has occurred and egg release can be expected within 24-44 hours), the woman can schedule an ultrasound exam and the insemination for the next day, if possible.

It is very important to be examined via ultrasound prior to the insemination, since urine tests that predict ovulation can be misleading, difficult to read, or incorrect. For instance, the urine test could show a positive result on day 12 of a woman's cycle, but her ultrasound exam might show her follicles to be only 15 mm in size. This would mean that the urine test has given a false positive, which occasionally occurs in patients who have been treated with clomiphene. Since follicles grow approximately 2 mm per day and the target size for maturity is 20 mm, the doctor could predict that the insemination should take place four days later. The timing of the actual insemination procedure is important, but not critical. Since the best time for fertilization is 24-48 hours after the LH surge, insemination should ideally take place during the day following the positive urine test—provided the ultrasound confirms that the test did not produce a false positive. But since pregnancy can result from exposure to sperm any time from four days prior to the actual ovulation to 18 hours afterwards, if the LH surge occurs on a Saturday evening and the doctor's office is closed on Sunday, Monday morning will not be too late for the insemination. Waiting any longer than 54 hours after the LH surge is risky, since the eggs will start to deteriorate and the cervical mucus will dry up beginning around 18 hours after their release.

SUCCESS RATES FOR IUI + CLOMIPHENE CITRATE

The combination of IUI and clomiphene citrate should be successful within three treatment cycles. Nearly 85% of all pregnancies that occur with this treatment will take place during the first six months; 65% of those will take place during the first three cycles. Repeated treatments beyond three to four cycles will be wasteful, unproductive and frustrating. Thus, if you and your partner don't achieve a pregnancy after three months of clomiphene plus IUI, you should be prepared to proceed to the next level of treatment.

CLINICAL CASE STUDY:
CLOMIPHENE CITRATE + IUI: DONNA AND FRANK

Donna (37-years-old) and Frank (40-years-old) had a four-year-old son who had been conceived naturally after only four months of trying. On their son's second birthday, the couple decided it was time to provide him with a sibling. Since the first conception had been so easy, they didn't expect any problems. But when Donna still hadn't become pregnant after nearly two years of well-timed intercourse, they decided to seek medical help.

Donna's basic fertility evaluation seemed to be normal and she had a low FSH level (10). However, her egg reserve was low, with only two to three primary follicles per section examined. Frank was found to have a high sperm count, but the motility before processing was lower than normal.

During their first cycle of clomiphene plus IUI, Donna was given 100 mg per day of the medication on days 2 to 7 of her cycle. She produced only two follicles and did not conceive. To improve her response, the doctor increased Donna's clomiphene to 150 mg/day for seven days, but for this cycle she produced only a single follicle. A sonogram showed her endometrium to be thin and her cervical mucus to be scant, due to the effects of the medication. Not surprisingly, the IUI was again unsuccessful.

The doctor diagnosed Donna's problem as egg depletion—even though she was not yet "officially" premenopausal. Her few remaining oocytes were likely to be of poor genetic quality; therefore, the doctor suspected that Donna might not be able to conceive. The fact that Donna had low ovarian reserve and responded poorly to clomiphene indicated that she would probably not respond well even to high doses of more potent, injectable fertility drugs. Donna and her husband were informed of this possibility, yet elected to try a course of high-dose injectable fertility medications (step # 2 in *The Pregnancy Prescription*). Having taken the maximum dosage of injectable medications, Donna still only produced two follicles and did not conceive.

According to their physician, continuing to the next level of infertility treatment, IVF, would not help this couple achieve a pregnancy. Oocyte quality issues resulting from an age factor are not successfully treated by IVF. Furthermore, the use of high doses of injectable fertility drugs would not be helpful, since she would not be expected to produce significantly more egg follicles with injectable drugs than the single follicle that she produced each month without medication. Therefore, Donna and Frank were strongly advised against trying IVF or the continued use of injectable medications. The couple was presented with three realistic options:

1. They could continue trying to conceive on their own, naturally, in the hope that Donna still had "a few good eggs," one of which would create a pregnancy.
2. They could try to conceive using donor eggs.
3. They could adopt.

In this couple's situation, IVF or any other form of fertility-enhancing therapy are not "magic bullets" that can be used to treat all forms of infertility problems successfully. Ultimately, natural selection and genetics will determine when and if conception is to occur. Although Donna and Frank were heartbroken over their prognosis, the success-oriented approach saved them time, money and future disappointments in their quest to have a baby.

SUMMARY

If a woman's Fallopian tubes are both open yet a couple has been unable to conceive due to a mild sperm problem, irregular or infrequent ovulation, or unexplained infertility, the combination of clomiphene citrate plus IUI offers a safe, cost-effective, first step towards conception. Increasing the number of eggs and putting more sperm near them at the time of ovulation is the easiest way to enhance the natural process of conception. Twenty to thirty percent of couples will conceive at this initial stage of treatment.

Clomiphene may not work for everyone, but it can give a good indication of the ovaries' ability to produce multiple egg follicles. Generally, the better the egg reserve, the better a woman's response to all fertility drugs, so that a basic "rule of thumb" is that the more eggs that can be produced, the better a woman's chances of conceiving. Of course, there are exceptions to every rule, but in cases in which there is low ovarian reserve, the number of follicles produced will be low, even in response to high doses of the most potent fertility drugs.

If your response to clomiphene is a good one, but you have not conceived after three cycles of treatment, do not despair. Your prognosis is still favorable for becoming pregnant and you should plan to move on to the next step, described in Chapter 6.

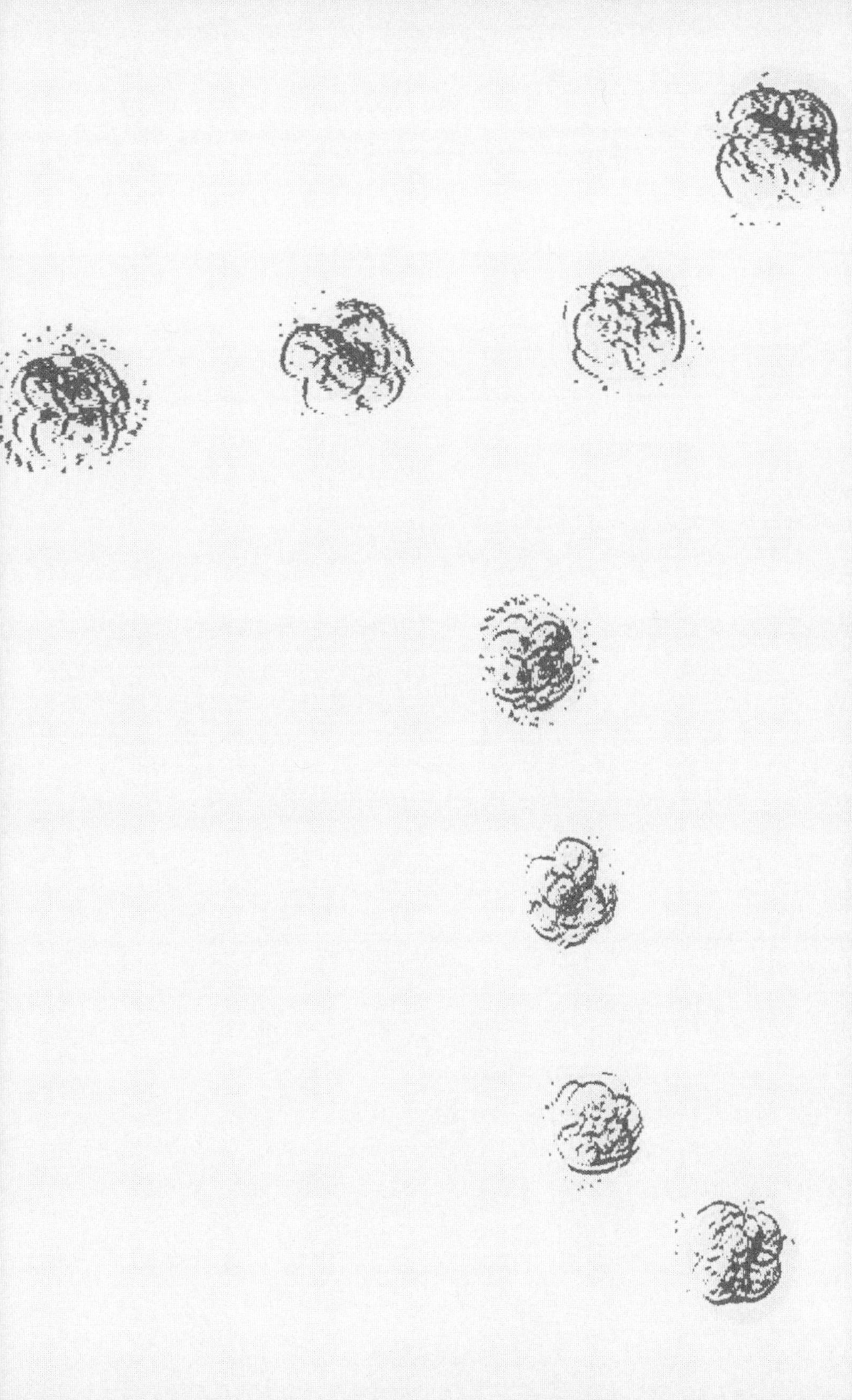

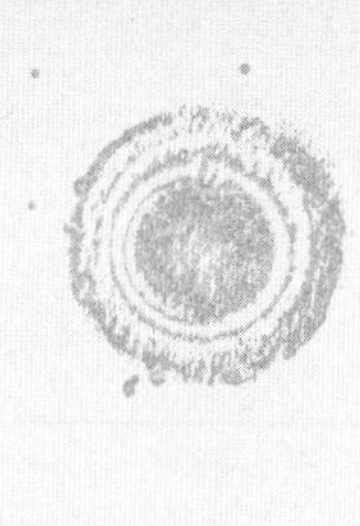
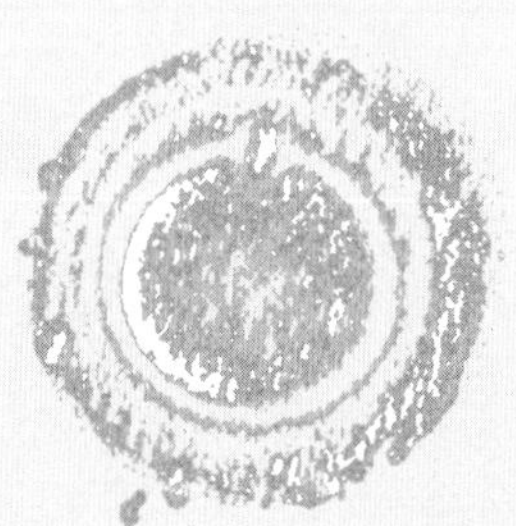
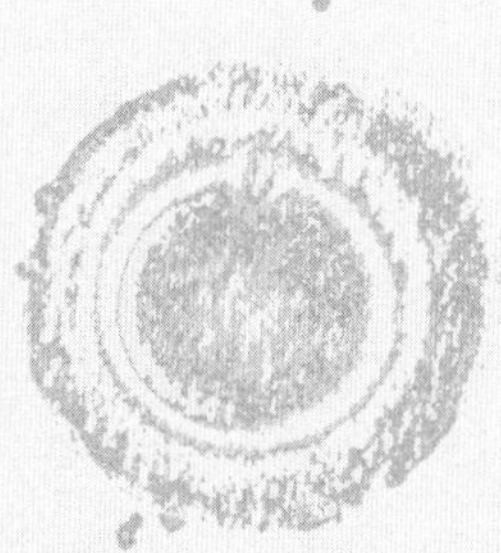
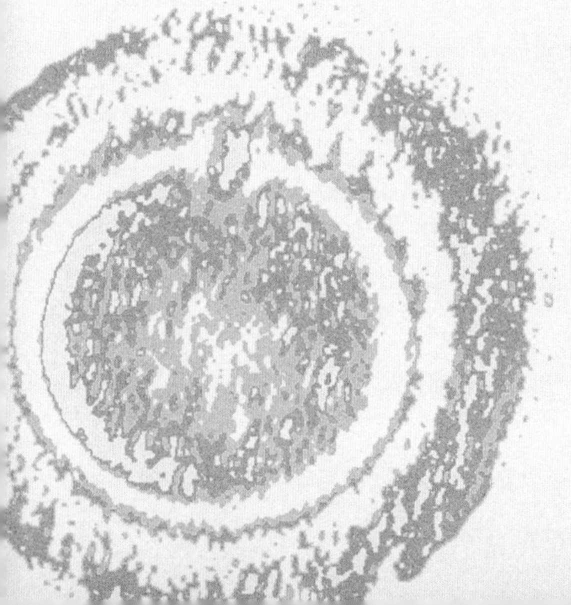

CHAPTER 6

STEP 2

The Treatment of Infertility Injectable Fertility Drugs and Intrauterine Insemination (IUI)

If you have not ovulated while taking oral medications or have had three unsuccessful cycles with the combination of clomiphene citrate and Intrauterine Insemination (IUI), your next step might be to move to a combination of more potent fertility drugs and IUI.

You might be an especially good candidate for this next step under the following conditions:

- If you produced little or thick cervical mucus or a thin endometrium when you were taking oral medications
- If both of your Fallopian tubes are open
- If your post-coital test (PCT) shows few or absent sperm in the cervical mucus, although your partner's sperm count is fairly normal

However, you might consider skipping this step and proceeding directly to IVF treatment if any of the following conditions prevails:

- One of your Fallopian tubes is blocked
- The sonogram shows endometriomas (masses of endometrial tissue in your ovaries)
- You have a good PCT
- The sperm specimen consistently has a count of less than 5 million motile sperm

GONADOTROPINS: THE "HEAVY HITTERS" OF FERTILITY DRUGS

Gonadotropins are injectable fertility drugs that, when the ovarian reserve is good, induce a woman to produce an even greater number of follicles than clomiphene citrate. Where clomiphene stimulates the hypothalamus (the ovulation control center in the brain) and affects the ovary only indirectly, gonadotropins act directly on the ovaries to provide a greater number of eggs for the sperm to fertilize.

Gonadotropin therapy must be highly individualized, since no two patients will respond to the drug in exactly the same manner. It requires a great deal of experience on the part of the physician to produce an optimal amount of follicles for each patient without overshooting or undershooting the mark. Factors such as age, body mass, menstrual history and ovarian follicular reserve determine both the starting dosage and necessary frequency of monitoring. The purpose of the therapy—whether it is for ovulation induction only or for IUI or *In Vitro* Fertilization (IVF)—also determines a physician's approach to a patient's therapeutic regimen. For example, a young woman who does not get her period and has enlarged ovaries with a very high egg reserve will be initially treated with very low doses of gonadotropins and be monitored frequently. That is because such patients are usually overly responsive to these drugs and are at high risk for ovarian hyperstimulation and multiple births, especially with IUI. If such a patient were undergoing IUI therapy, a lower dosage would be prescribed than if she were to undergo IVF; too many eggs are not desirable for IUI in younger patients, whereas relatively higher numbers of eggs are obviously advantageous for IVF. In the case of a 38-year-old woman with a high egg reserve and regular periods, the situation is quite different. Such a patient is neither at risk for ovarian hyperstimulation nor multiple births. Rather, a higher degree of stimulation would be greatly advantageous, since with advanced age, relatively few eggs are genetically competent enough to result in a normal pregnancy.

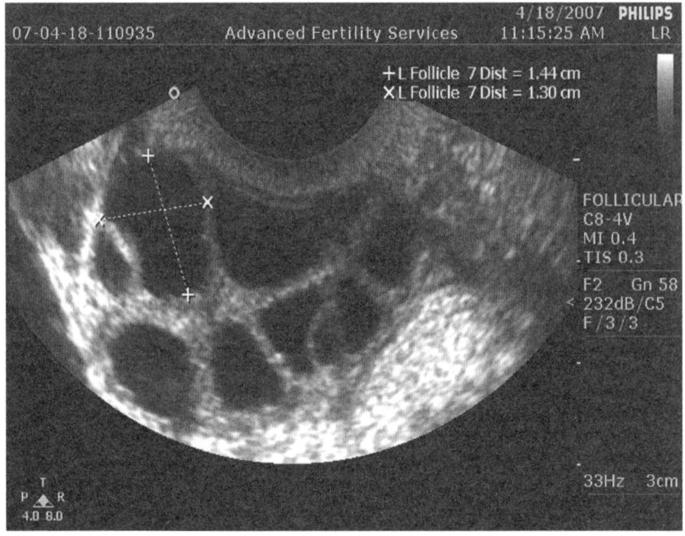

Fig. 1. ***Multiple egg follicles induced by the injection of gonadotropins. Note that the response is much greater than with Clomid (refer to Chapter 5 Fig. 1.)***

WHICH ONE TO CHOOSE?

When a patient is undergoing IUI therapy with injectable medications, the currently available gonadotropins—Follistim, Gonal-F, Menopur, Repronex and Bravelle—are basically similar, the major ingredient being FSH, which is the body's natural hormone that is responsible for egg development. Generally, patients who respond well to one drug will respond in a similar fashion to another. Likewise, if a woman produces very few follicles with one gonadotropin, she will respond equally poorly to all others. From a practical standpoint, the major difference between the gonadotropins is that Follistim and Gonal-F are administered with a premixed cartridge and pen system, whereas Bravelle and Menopur need to be mixed prior to injection with a syringe. All use a tiny needle and are injected subcutaneously. Each of these medications has certain advantages. For patients who are anxious about mixing medications and injecting themselves, the simplicity of using the cartridge system has great appeal. Yet an ingenious mixing device has facilitated the use of Bravelle and Menopur. An advantage of using Bravelle and Menopur is that other medications, such as Lupron, can be added to it, thereby eliminating one injection per day. The individual gonadotropins and their unique usages, as well as their potential major complication, the Ovarian Hyperstimulation Syndrome, will be discussed in detail in Chapter 7.

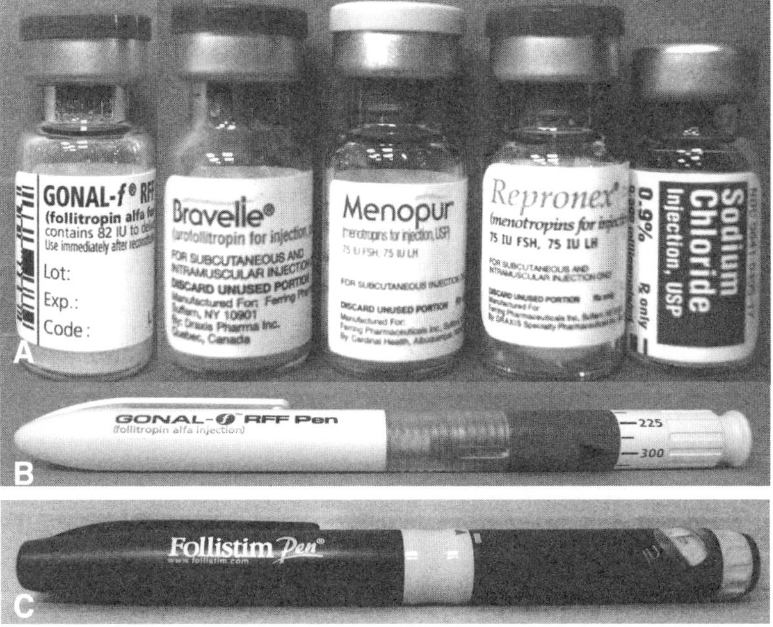

Fig. 2. *Currently available gonadotropins.*
A. *Mixable forms of FSH. Although they involve some preparation, they have the advantage of being able to mix multiple medications, including Lupron, in a single injection.*
B. & C. *Pen injection systems require no mixing and are easier to use. They cannot have other medications mixed with them, so multiple injections are required when they are used in most treatment protocols.*

HOW GONADOTROPINS ARE USED

Treating patients with injectable drugs is an art, much like the creation of fine cuisine. A good chef doesn't merely follow a recipe from a cookbook, but modifies it depending on the individual ingredients available at the time. Just as the taste and flavor of fresh ingredients vary greatly from season to season, so do patients vary in their responses to the medications. Rather than take a "cookbook" approach to patients, a physician must consider a multitude of factors when creating an ovarian stimulation protocol for a particular patient. Unfortunately, all too often the selection of a stimulation protocol is determined solely by the patient's age, based on the unfounded assumption that all younger patients will be good responders. Other important factors, such as weight, menstrual history, ovarian reserve and hormonal status, must also be factored into the treatment equation. Of all factors that need to be considered, I believe that the ovarian reserve is the most important in formulating the initial stimulation protocol.

In regularly menstruating women, injectable fertility medications are always started very early in the menstrual cycle, usually on day 2, 3 or 4. By cycle day 5, a single dominant follicle has already been selected, so that any other follicles that will develop will be "late bloomers" and will not reach maturity by the time the dominant follicle is ready for fertilization.

Obviously, the creation of multiple immature eggs is not desirable for successful treatment. However, if a woman's ovulatory cycle is naturally longer than 28 days, stimulation can be started at a correspondingly later time. For example, if the normal cycle is every 34 days, ovulation occurs around day 20. Consequently, the dominant follicle would not be selected until day nine or ten, so the stimulation can be started by cycle day 8 or 9. Patients who do not get their periods can begin their stimulation at any time as long as the endometrium is thin. If the endometrium is thick, it must be cleaned off by a course of progesterone prior to stimulation in order to have the lining of the uterus be in sync for possible embryo implantation.

The medication protocol must be monitored in order to determine the optimal time of egg maturity and the number of eggs that can potentially be formed, as well as to prevent the ovarian hyperstimulation syndrome. The monitoring schedule for a patient's stimulation protocol with blood tests and sonograms should also be individualized, so that it is effective without being burdensome. The most important concept to note is that patients who are high responders need to be monitored more frequently than low-responding patients. This is necessary in order to prevent over stimulation and an unacceptably high rate of multiple pregnancies in high-responding patients. Intermediate or low-responding patients are at virtually no risk for ovarian overstimulation.

Daily monitoring throughout the entire stimulation protocol is unnecessary, except possibly in the last few days of higher-responding patients' treatment protocols. Physicians understand that visits to the IVF center for blood tests and sonograms are time consuming and stressful, causing time lost from work, unusual fatigue from lost sleep due to early-morning appointments required by many clinics (6-7 a.m.) and the discomfort of repeated venapuncture. Being sensitive to this, physicians usually try to have a patient come for monitoring as infrequently as possible without sacrificing the safety and efficacy of the treatment. In addition, there is usually some degree of flexibility for monitoring, depending on the day that the stimulation is started. So be sure to inform your doctor if there is some conflict in your schedule such as an important business meeting or a short business trip that cannot be postponed. It will usually be possible to make the necessary adjustments in your monitoring schedule to accommodate your needs. Recognizing that some degree of flexibility is possible will reduce the amount of stress that is experienced when scheduling conflicts arise.

MONITORING A STIMULATION CYCLE

Whether a stimulation protocol is used for IUI or IVF, the monitoring is quite similar at the beginning. All patients should have a baseline sonogram to eliminate the possibility of new or previously existing ovarian cysts, which could interfere with stimulation or confuse the interpretation of subsequent sonograms. Also, the endometrial lining should be seen to be thin and clear so that it can thicken to a point that it is ready to receive an embryo at the appropriate time. The FSH, LH and estradiol levels must also be checked to ensure that the patient responds properly to the stimulation. Ideally, they should all be low; the lower, the better. If there is a functioning ovarian cyst or if the blood tests are elevated the cycle will not be started, since egg follicle development will assuredly not proceed as it should. When this occurs, the physician will either postpone the start of the cycle or cancel it, while taking steps to remedy the situation so that treatment can be resumed in a subsequent cycle.

The next visit for monitoring would be—at the earliest—after three days of injections and—at the latest, following five or six days of treatment. A young or very thin patient, a patient with a high ovarian reserve, or a woman with polycystic ovarian syndrome will require earlier and more frequent monitoring than older patients and those with lower levels of ovarian reserve. After the first monitoring results are known, the patient is usually monitored every two to three days until the largest follicles are in the range of an average diameter between 16-20 mm. More recently, we have been able to calculate the volume of each ovarian follicle that has been stimulated and have determined that any follicle with a volume over 2.00 cubic mm will contain a mature oocyte. When the follicles reach a size that contain eggs that are capable of taking the final steps to maturity, the patient is ready for HCG, the final—and most important—injection of the cycle. For example, a 28-year-old woman, weighing 105 lbs., who never gets a period without medication would be started on a very low dose of FSH—perhaps 50 units per day. After three days of treatment, if there is no rise in the estradiol level the dosage could be raised very minimally to 75 units per day for three more days. Since the patient is having an IUI cycle, it is not desirable to produce too many follicles. Therefore, the dosage would be kept at the same minimal level for another three days and then, if the estradiol level doesn't budge, the dose might be increased slightly—to 100 units on a daily basis. Once the estradiol level starts to move upwards, the sonogram will show slight growth in the average follicular size and an increase in the thickness of the endometrium. At this time, the ovaries are starting to respond, and the patient must be monitored every 24-48 hours so she does not overshoot the mark. This would necessitate the cancellation of the cycle. Unfortunately, with the first treatment cycle, it is impossible to know the extent of a patient's sensitivity to the injectables. Therefore, some patients' stimulation will progress slowly while others may have their estrogen levels shoot up precipitously, producing an excess of follicles and causing cycle cancellation.

In both instances, it is natural for patients to experience a considerable amount of frustration and disappointment. It is important to remember that each patient varies in her response to these medications and, based on objective information (history and age, body weight, ovarian reserve and hormonal levels) and clinical experience from treating many patients, the doctor can only make an "educated guess" in determining the starting point of an individual's therapy. If the initial approach does not produce the desired stimulation, the next cycle should be improved as a result of what is learned from your previously unsuccessful response.

Another clinical example is that of a 38-year-old woman who wishes to have a second child. She weighs 186 lbs. and has a moderate ovarian reserve. In this situation, because of her weight, advanced age and the presence of only a moderate reserve of follicles, this patient would need much higher doses of FSH (300-450 units per day) to stimulate multiple follicles. Because she is older and has fewer follicles in reserve, she is neither at significant risk for ovarian hyperstimulation nor of multiple birth. After making sure baseline studies were normal, her initial monitoring appointment would be after five to six days of treatment, when the follicles would be expected to be near mature size. In this woman's case, monitoring would be necessary only for the determination of egg maturity and the subsequent timing of the HCG injection.

HCG AND THE WINDOW OF FERTILIZATION

When the follicles are in the appropriate size range and the estradiol levels are not too elevated, the patient is ready to receive an HCG injection. This will complete the process of egg maturation—a process that takes between 28 and 42 hours to complete and ends with the rupture of the ovarian follicle and the release of a mature egg.

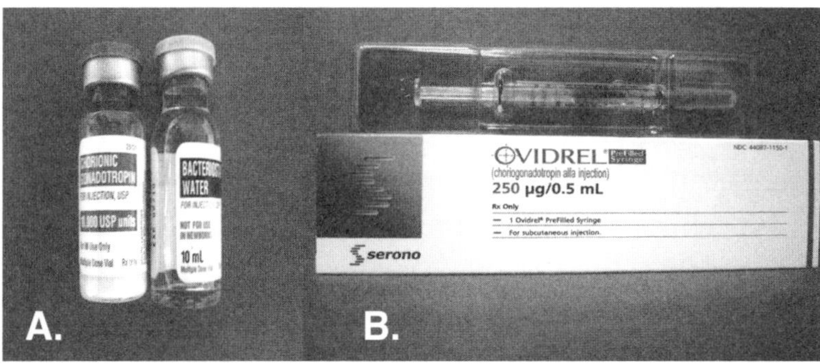

Fig. 3. ***Types of HCG that are used.***
A. This HCG preparation is the traditional form of the medication which must be mixed prior to injection. This medication must be given with a larger needle into the muscle. There is also the possibility of error when mixing this medication which would result in the failure of egg development. Extreme care must be employed so that the water vial is not confused with the vial of active medication.
B. Ovidrel is the new form of HCG which is premixed and given subcutaneously with a very small needle. I prefer using this form of the medication since it is virtually error proof in administration and is much less painful for the patients.

The actual window of fertilization begins with the HCG injection and ends approximately 12 hours after the follicle ruptures, which is a period of nearly 60 hours. Since spermatozoa can stay alive in the woman's reproductive tract at the time of ovulation for 24-96 hours, sexual intercourse or insemination occurring during that time interval could cause fertilization.

Some of the greatest concerns that patients express to me relate to the timing and frequency of intercourse or insemination during the window of fertilization. Many people incorrectly assume that the sperm must be introduced at the exact moment of ovulation, when the egg releases from the ovarian follicle. The truth is that sperm can live in the female reproductive tract for many days, as long as the mucus in the female reproductive tract is as it should be during the ovulatory period. An example of this is a case that occurred in the 1950s, in which a woman gave birth to a set of fraternal twins who looked very much like two different gentlemen with whom the mother had been simultaneously involved. Although DNA testing was not available at the time, simple blood typing proved that there were two different males involved in the twins' conception. The woman admitted to having intercourse with both men, with a seven-day interval between the sex acts. This is a memorable example of how long sperm can wait to meet an egg in the female reproductive tract.

Since conception is a natural process, it is crucial to remember that we, as individuals, have little control over it other than enjoying making love on an occasional basis. Conception will either happen or not, depending on genetic factors that occur around the time of fertilization. The frequency of sexual intercourse, whether it occurs on a daily or alternate day basis, the sexual positions employed or the fact that a woman rests on her back with her legs elevated, has no impact on conception. Likewise, IUI can be performed any time between 24 and 48 hours after an HCG injection. If the sperm count is high, with over 20 million active sperm, one IUI should be more than adequate for fertilization. In the event that the number of active sperm is low, insemination on two consecutive days may be beneficial in increasing the total number of sperm in the woman's reproductive system. Although the number of active sperm required to cause a pregnancy naturally with sexual intercourse is not known, I have had patients occasionally conceive with as few as 2 million active sperm in the insemination specimen.

In an injectable cycle, a spontaneous LH surge rarely occurs. Therefore, HCG is mandatory to complete egg maturation and release. Typically, if HCG were given on a Saturday evening between 6 and 9 p.m., the IUI would be scheduled for Monday. Usually, the follicles will rupture by late that afternoon. At that time the oocyte, along with the fluid contents of the follicle, is expelled and settles in the deepest area in the pelvis, the so-called "pouch of Douglas." Follicular release is visualized sonographically, showing collapsed follicles and an accumulation of follicular fluid in the floor of the pelvis. The mop-like ends of the Fallopian tubes naturally fall into the pouch of Douglas, so that when oocytes are released into that area, the egg—surrounded by a sticky ring of cells, called cumulus cells—adheres to the fimbria and are drawn into the Fallopian tube, ready to meet with the patiently waiting spermatozoa. As long as follicular fluid is seen in the pelvis, the egg is still fertilizable.

Once the fluid is no longer present—about 12 hours after follicle rupture—the window of fertility is closed.

WHEN EGGS DON'T RELEASE

When several follicles are stimulated with fertility drugs, not all follicles rupture at the same time. In fact, about 15% of the time follicles may not rupture at all. This is called the Luteinized Unreleased Follicle Syndrome. Typically, all conventional tests indicate ovulation has occurred, but pregnancy cannot result because the egg remains stuck within the follicle and cannot come in contact with the sperm. The diagnosis is made sonographically, when a follow-up study shows an intact follicle and absence of fluid in the pelvis 60 hours after the HCG injection. This phenomenon rarely occurs in normally ovulating women, but is a frequent occurrence in women who are said to have the Polycystic Ovary Syndrome. This is because the ovaries of these patients have a thickened capsule, which makes follicle rupture more difficult.

If the majority of follicles consistently fail to rupture, a procedure called Follicular Puncture with Intraperitoneal Insemination can be employed as an alternative to IVF. In Follicular Puncture, the physician removes the woman's entrapped mature eggs directly from her ovaries with an ultrasound-guided needle and deposits them in the pouch of Douglas where they would normally accumulate after ovulation. Then, with the needle still in place, the doctor injects her partner's processed sperm into the same space. This places egg and sperm in as close proximity as possible, hopefully enhancing the chances for fertilization. This procedure, though a viable alternative in the past when the

IVF success rates were not as good as they are currently, is used infrequently today. To a great extent, this is also due to the fact that the procedure is not covered by insurance. However, Follicular Puncture is used to help couples that, because of religious belief, cannot undergo IVF treatment, since fertilization is natural and occurs within the human body rather than in a laboratory.

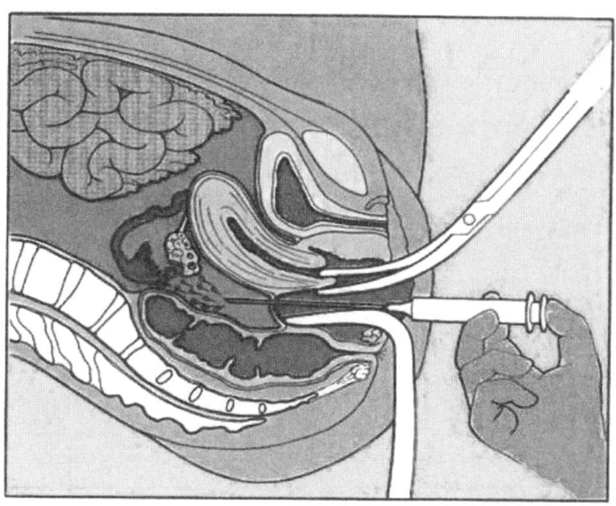

Fig. 4. ***The technique of intraperitoneal insemination, illustrating where the egg and sperm most probably meet in the body at the time of fertilization.***

There have been no reported cases of abdominal implantation of embryos created via IPI, although theoretically this could be possible since fertilization takes place inside the body but outside the Fallopian tube.

SUCCESS RATES

As long as a woman has at least one open (patent) tube, approximately 20% of couples will conceive within three cycles of gonadotropins combined with IUI. If the couple does not achieve a pregnancy after a maximum of three treatment cycles, they should move on to IVF.

Of the couples that undergo IVF after failing to conceive with IUI, 35-75% can be expected to become pregnant after several IVF cycles. Many of these couples will turn out to have fertilization problems that could only have been detected via IVF.

CLINICAL CASE STUDY
GONADOTROPINS + IUI:
PATRICIA AND SAM

Pat (33-years-old) and Sam (32-years-old) had been trying to conceive for three years. Pat's evaluation showed no obvious reason for her failure to become pregnant. Her blood test for antichlamydia antibodies was negative, and her tubes appeared to be open. Ultrasound exams showed her to be ovulating.

Semen analysis indicated that Sam had a "borderline" specimen, with sperm that was classified as "subnormal" with respect to shape and motility. For that reason, the doctor decided to help Nature along with a trial of clomiphene citrate and IUI. Pat responded well to the medication and produced four to six follicles during each of three cycles, but the couple still didn't conceive.

Pat and Sam then moved on to Step 2. Pat was instructed to take 300 units of Follistim on cycle days 2 and 3 of her next cycle, and then 2 amps per day thereafter, until day 10. When Pat saw the doctor for monitoring on day 11, he discovered that she had produced 10 mature-sized follicles. He advised her to take HCG that evening, and an IUI was performed with 10 million motile sperm on cycle day 13, 36 hours later. Two weeks later, Pat had the wonderful news that she was pregnant. Four weeks after an insemination, an ultrasound showed a single gestational sac in the uterus. Utilizing the process described as Step 2 of *The Pregnancy Prescription* to facilitate the meeting of multiple eggs with a high concentration of sperm, the natural process of fertilization was augmented and fortunately resulted in a pregnancy. Pat and Sam were indeed fortunate to have conceived. If Pat was several years older or had poor ovarian reserve, their story might not have ended on such a happy note.

S U M M A R Y

The injectable fertility drugs known as gonadotropins can help a woman produce greater numbers of mature eggs than clomiphene citrate, without any of the negative effects associated with the oral agents. Patients who do not conceive after three cycles of oral agents combined with IUI are at a critical juncture in their decision-making process regarding the direction of future treatment. A patient with normal Fallopian tubes and poor post-coital tests would be advised to proceed to the next step in *The Pregnancy Prescription*, using gonadotropins and IUI. A patient who has one blocked Fallopian tube and a normal post-coital test would probably not receive any benefit from Step 2 and should proceed directly to IVF. Those patients with a poor egg follicle response to both oral and injectable medications should not pursue IVF, but rather consider egg donation or adoption.

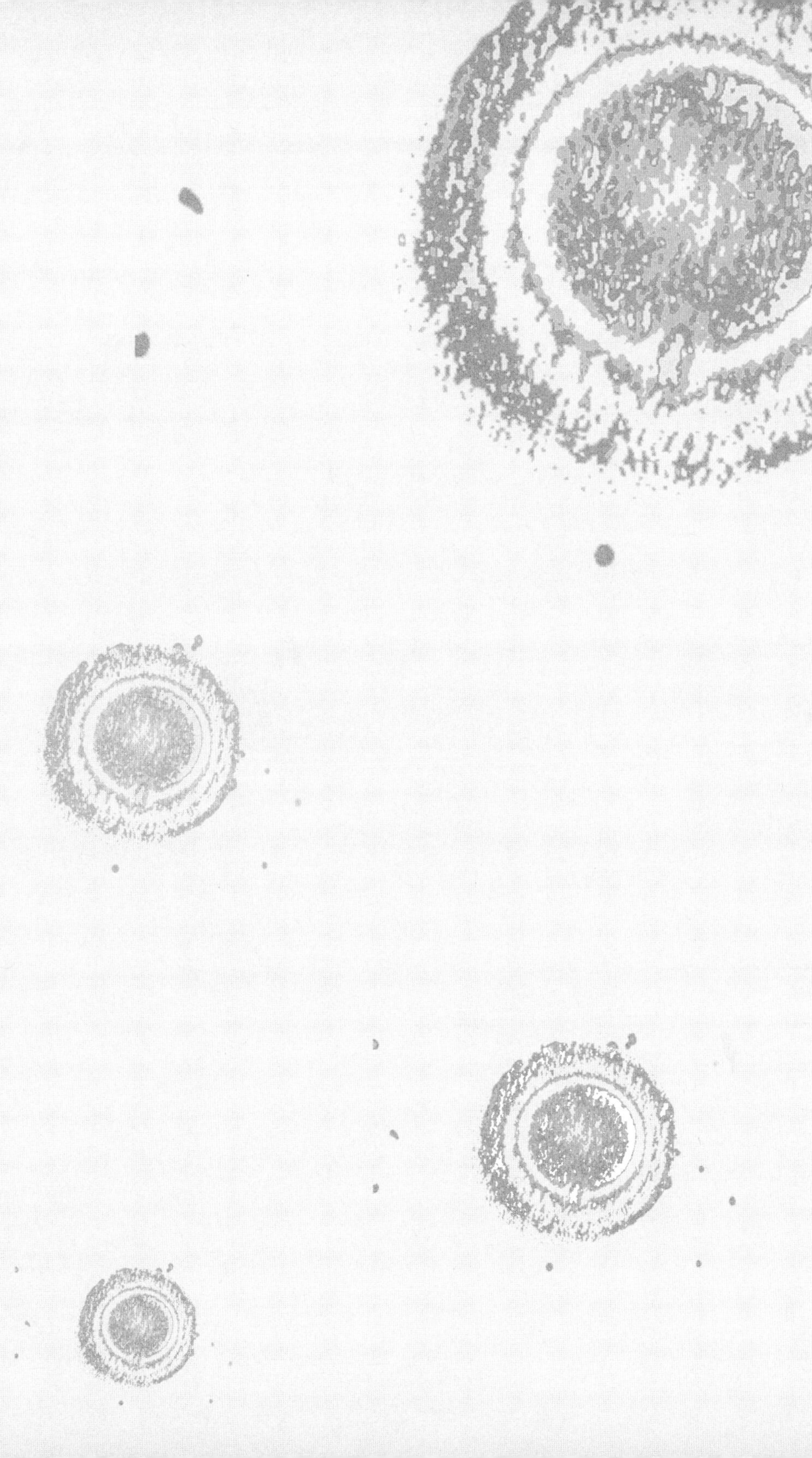

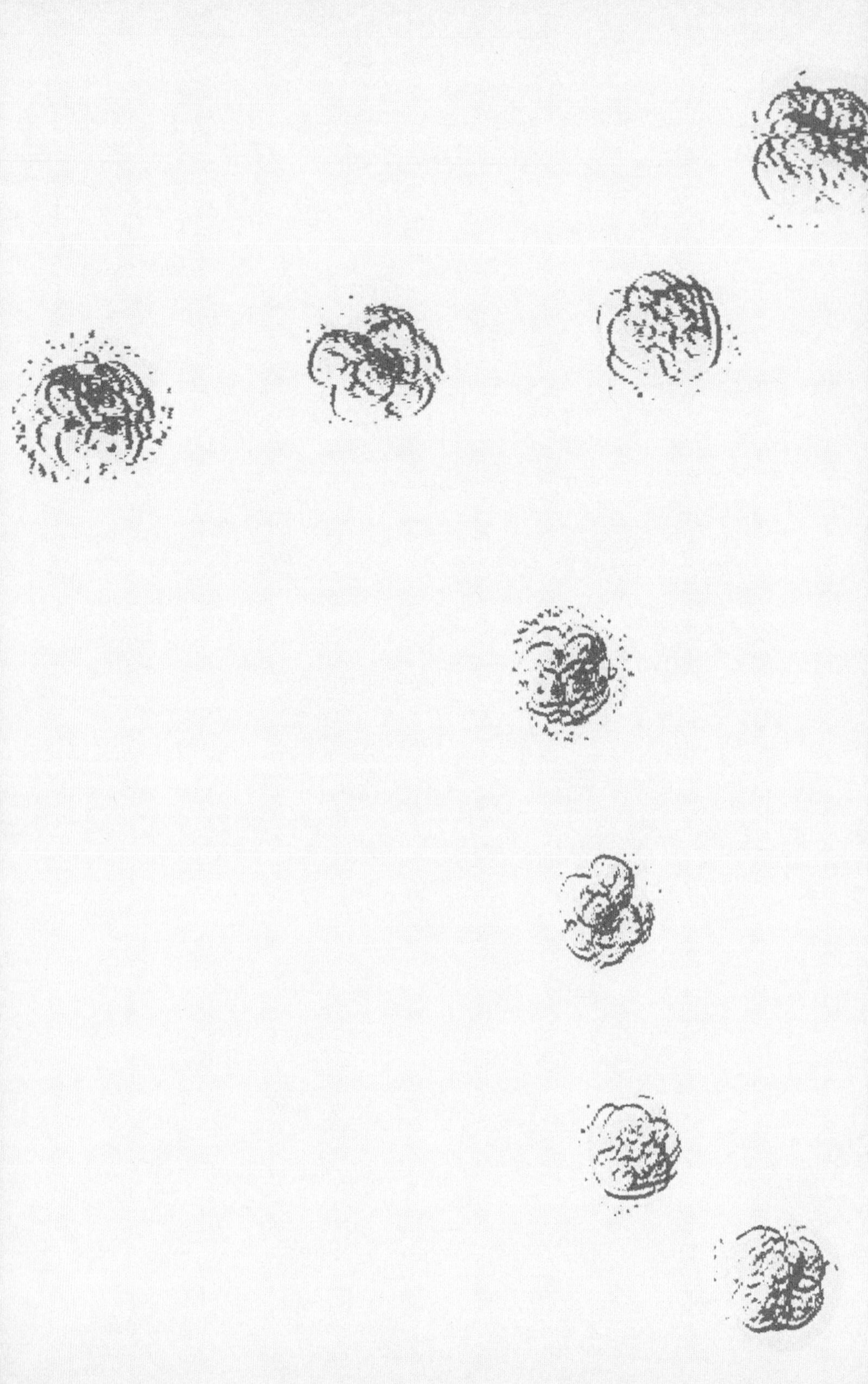

CHAPTER 7

STEP 3

In Vitro Fertilization Stimulation Protocols

If you have already undergone treatment with gonadotropins + Intrauterine Insemination (IUI) without becoming pregnant, you are probably feeling discouraged. Don't lose hope. You still have a good chance of conceiving the child you want so desperately—but in your case, nature may need some extra help from modern technology.

If you have not conceived after a maximum of six cycles of fertility drugs combined with insemination, *In Vitro* Fertilization (IVF) should be your next step in *The Pregnancy Prescription.* However, couples that have been diagnosed with any of the following may want to *begin* their fertility treatment with IVF:

- Extremely poor sperm quality: sperm count of less than 5 million after processing; velocity (speed) of less than 60 mic/second after processing; and/or very poor morphology (shape)
- Both Fallopian tubes completely blocked
- One Fallopian tube blocked *plus* testing positive for anti-chlamydial antibodies
- A previous history of ectopic pregnancy and failure to conceive after at least one year of unprotected intercourse
- Severe endometriosis, with or without a history of surgery
- Long-standing (three to four years), unexplained infertility—particularly if the woman is in her mid-30s

A typical IVF cycle includes the following phases:

1. Stimulation of egg follicles
2. Monitoring of follicle development
3. Oocyte retrieval
4. Fertilization
5. Embryo transfer

OVARIAN STIMULATION

To maximize the chances for a successful IVF cycle, a physician will use drugs to stimulate the ovaries to produce large numbers of eggs that will mature at approximately the same rate. Medications to be used and how to use them will be based on the individual characteristics of each patient, as well as the physician's personal experience. A drug protocol is the general form of stimulation used for the induction of ovulation or for controlled ovarian hyperstimulation for IUI or IVF. Drug protocols also refer to the specific treatment schedule that your doctor designs for your IVF cycle, comprising the specific medications used, their dosage and the timing of their administration. We have already discussed the gonadotropins in Chapter 6. In this chapter, I will begin by describing the role of Leuprolide acetate (Lupron), another key drug used in IVF treatment regimens. I will also describe different ways in which these drugs are used in IVF. These protocols are usually quite different from those used for IUI cycles.

LEUPROLIDE ACETATE (LUPRON)

Lupron is a class of drug called an agonist, which is used to suppress the normal monthly production of a single egg. This function is important, as it enables the natural process of ovulation to be overridden so that multiple egg follicles can be stimulated in a uniform manner. In the IVF procedure, it is critical that the eggs reach maturity at approximately the same time, since a woman's eggs need to be at exactly the right stage of maturity in their development when they are exposed to the sperm. Fertilization can occur only during the stage known as Metaphase II—the point at which the number of chromosomes contained in the egg drops from 46 to 23. If Metaphase II has not yet occurred at the time of the IVF retrieval, the eggs will contain too much genetic material (46 chromosomes) and will either be unable to become fertilized or produce an abnormal embryo containing excess genetic material.

Lupron is also essential in the IVF process since its use prevents the spontaneous release of the eggs from the ovarian follicles prior to egg retrieval. The premature rupture of the follicles and the subsequent loss of the eggs will necessitate the termination of the treatment cycle.

A disadvantage of Lupron is that some women taking this drug will not develop their egg follicles properly, in a timely fashion. This condition is called ovarian oversuppression. In general, women with diminished ovarian reserve, especially those in their late 30s, do not respond well to Lupron.

Lupron can be administered in various dosages and at various times in the menstrual cycle, depending on the patient's individual characteristics and on her unique pattern of ovarian response. The two most common dosing regimens are the "Long Lupron" (started seven days after ovulation) and the "Flare" (started during the menstrual period) protocols.

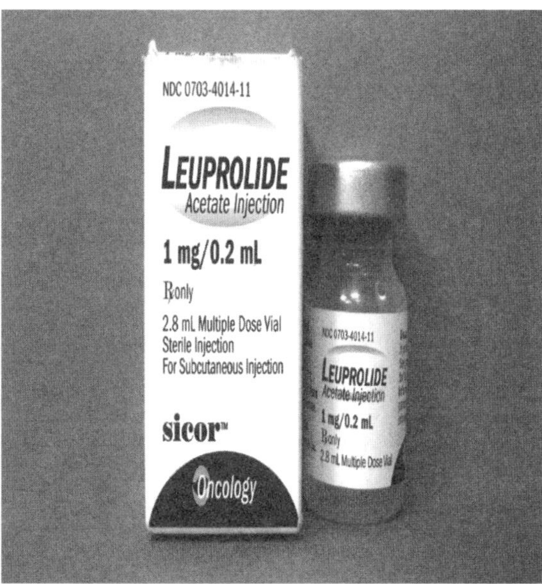

Fig. 1. ***Lupron is given subcutaneously with a very tiny needle. At current daily dosage levels of 5-10 units/day, a medication kit will last for 30 days.***

Long Lupron Protocol

With this regimen, the woman begins taking her Lupron injections during the last week of the menstrual cycle that precedes the start of her IVF cycle. The purpose of starting the injections at this time is to prevent the next month's eggs from beginning to be stimulated, since eggs are actually "recruited" for a particular cycle during the one that precedes it. This ensures that the only eggs developed for the IVF cycle are those stimulated via the FSH injections.

Flare Protocol

With this regimen, used mainly for women who do not respond well to ovarian stimulation, the administration of Lupron begins on cycle day 2 to 3 of the woman's IVF cycle. This regimen generally has the opposite effect of the "Long Lupron" protocol in that, given *early* in the menstrual cycle, Lupron tends to cause an outpouring of FSH and LH from the pituitary gland before it begins to suppress the production of these hormones. A variation on the Flare protocol—the "Microdose Flare"—has also been found to be useful for women who respond poorly to ovarian stimulation.

CUSTOMIZING MEDICATION PROTOCOLS FOR OPTIMAL RESULTS

To predict which medications are most likely to produce the best results, a doctor will evaluate each patient as to whether she is most likely to be a normal responder, low responder, or over responder. When it comes to prescribing fertility drugs, patients in each of these groups have their own special needs.

THE NORMAL RESPONDER

A woman in her 20s to mid-30s with a low FSH level on day 2 to 3 of her menstrual cycle and good ovarian reserve is considered to be a normal responder and will usually respond well to a "Day 21 Long Lupron regimen." The typical Day 21 Long Lupron protocol is illustrated in the following table. This example is based on a typical 28-day cycle.

Specific dosages of Lupron and FSH will vary, depending on how well the woman responds to the drug. The daily dosage of FSH may range from 2 to 8 ampules (150-600 units) per day. However, a patient who doesn't produce multiple follicles with 4 to 6 amps will rarely produce additional follicles despite an increased dose. Discontinuing Lupron—or changing to a different regimen—may cause such a woman to produce a greater number of egg follicles.

LONG LUPRON PROTOCOL		
BEGINNING ON DAY	**MEDICATION**	**ACTION**
21 of previous cycle	Lupron, 5-10 units/day	Stops naturally occurring egg development
2-3 of IVF cycle	Lupron, 2.5-5 units/day; start FSH	Start stimulation of multiple egg development
5-6 of IVF cycle	Adjust dose of Lupron and FSH	Continue egg stimulation; physician monitors blood levels and sonogram
9-10 of IVF cycle	Continue Lupron/adjust dose of FSH	Physician monitors blood tests and sonogram
11 of IVF cycle (if follicles are deemed mature)	Discontinue Lupron, FSH; take HCG at 9 p.m.	Starts the final stage of egg maturation
13 of IVF cycle—9 a.m. (36 hours later)		EGG RETRIEVAL

THE LOW RESPONDER

A woman with diminished ovarian reserve and FSH levels ranging from 10 to 15 mlU/ml on the second day of her cycle will usually not respond well to the day 21 Long Lupron protocol. These women generally do better with a Microdose Flare or a non-Lupron protocol. The European and Japanese Protocols are also appropriate for low responders. An example of the Microdose Flare Protocol is provided below.

BEGINNING ON DAY	MEDICATION	ACTION
2 of IVF cycle	Microdose Lupron; 6 amps of FSH	Egg stimulation
5 or 6 of IVF cycle	Continue Lupron and 6 amps of FSH	Physician monitors blood levels/sonogram
8-10 of IVF cycle	Adjust FSH dosage	Physician monitors blood tests/sonogram
11 of IVF cycle (or when follicles are deemed mature)	Discontinue Lupron and FSH; take HCG at 9 p.m.	Physician monitors blood tests/sonogram
13 of IVF cycle, 9 a.m.		EGG RETRIEVAL

THE PURE GONADOTROPIN PROTOCOL

Pure gonadotropin stimulation, without Lupron, is currently the most commonly employed protocol for low-responding patients and works equally well with normal responders. This approach has been made possible by the availability of the GnRH antagonist class of drugs, ganirelix acetate (Antagon) and cetrorelix actetate (Cetrotide). These drugs are used so that the stimulated follicles will not release their eggs prematurely, prior to egg retrieval. Most commonly, the antagonist is started when the follicles reach a diameter of 14 mm.

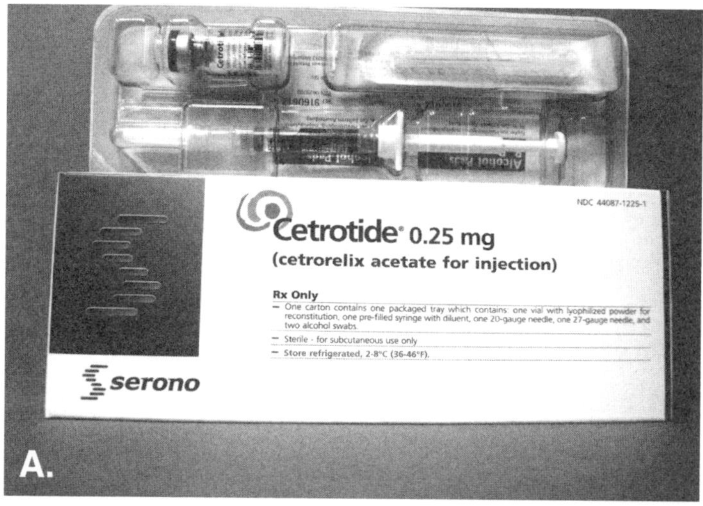

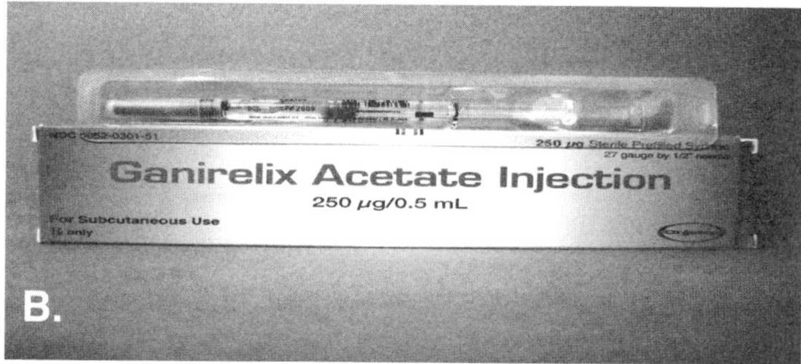

Fig. 2. A&B ***These drugs are called antagonists and are used to block an LH surge, which may occur prior to optimal egg development. They are administered subcutaneously with a very small needle.***

THE EUROPEAN PROTOCOL

I learned of this protocol, which is a potent stimulator of egg production, when I visited Hungary to attend a medical conference. This method was developed in Eastern European fertility clinics because the cost of drugs of the typical stimulation protocols was too high for their National Health Service budgets. Therefore, European fertility doctors developed a protocol combining Clomid and injectable FSH/LH, which was based on the original IVF stimulation regimens used in the late 1970s and early 1980s. The simultaneous combination of Clomid and FSH/LH, given on alternate days, yields a maximal response in terms of egg production, using many fewer injections and requiring approximately 50% less injectables, compared with the purely injectable regimens. Not only does this protocol save a great deal of money with respect to drug costs, it also greatly reduces the number of injections that a woman needs during a treatment cycle.

BCP x 21 days (last pill on a Thursday)

Sunday	Clomid 100 + 300 FSH
Monday	Clomid 100
Tuesday	Clomid 100 + 300 FSH
Wednesday	Clomid 100
Thursday	Clomid 100 + 300 FSH
Friday	300 FSH
Saturday	—
Sunday	—
Monday	Bloods and Sonogram/Possible HCG at 10 p.m.
Tuesday	—
Wednesday	Earliest Possible Retrieval

THE JAPANESE MINIMAL STIMULATION PROTOCOL

In Chapter 4, I discussed the "minimalist approach" to treating infertility and IVF stimulation. Proponents of minimal stimulation IVF believe that only a few high-quality eggs should be stimulated and harvested, with the goal of a single or dual embryo transfer. They cite several reasons for their approach. The most compelling reason is that this method virtually eliminates high-order multiple births by ensuring that there is not an excess number of embryos to transfer. The basis of their theory rests on the supposition that intense ovarian stimulation, which produces a great numbers of eggs, ultimately creates an excess of genetically abnormal embryos which are virtually indistinguishable from chromosomally perfect ones. In support of this theory is the fact that a surprisingly small percentage of normal-appearing embryos are found to be genetically perfect when subjected to genetic analysis. Since minimal stimulation is a very new concept, it remains to be seen whether this approach will prove beneficial for all patients or just certain subclasses of patients. To be sure, this method has certain advantages over traditional IVF stimulation in that it requires many fewer injections and less monitoring and should reduce the cost of an IVF cycle (less medication and fewer embryologic expenses). Moreover, the risks of ovarian hyperstimulation and high order multiple births are virtually nonexistent with the minimal stimulation protocol.

BEGINNING ON DAY	MEDICATION	ACTION
Start day 2 of IVF cycle	Start Clomid 50 mg/day	
Day 8	FSH 150 units	Sonogram every other day
Day 10	FSH 150 units (every other day)	
When largest follicle is 18mm and deemed mature	Stop Clomid and FSH; give HCG at 9 p.m.	Schedule egg retrieval 36 hours later

The European and Minimal Stimulation protocols are primarily useful in patients who are low responders. They are also ideal for patients who dread injections or have an aversion to high doses of fertility medications.

NATURAL IVF

As its name implies, Natural IVF is an unstimulated cycle. The goal of which is to retrieve the single mature egg created in a normal ovulatory cycle. The theoretical basis for advocating its usage is that the biologic process of natural selection will cause the highest-quality oocyte in the pool of eggs available for development in a given month to be contained in the dominant ovarian follicle. The trick is to carefully monitor the patients' cycle so as to retrieve the egg from the follicle when it is mature, but prior to follicular rupture and its release. In addition to monitoring follicle size via ultrasound (it should be 18-20 mm at maturity), careful attention must be paid to the LH levels. Once an LH surge has been detected in the blood, it is often impossible to predict when the patient will be in the narrow zone between egg maturity and its release. Scheduling the retrieval too early will result in the absence of an egg in the follicular fluid that is aspirated from the follicle, since if there is an insufficient time of exposure to LH, the oocyte will not complete its maturation and will not separate from the follicular wall. Yet if too much time is allowed for egg maturity, the egg will be released from the follicle prior to retrieval.

Fortunately, several strategies can be used to improve the chances of successful egg retrieval in Natural IVF. The most commonly used method is to give HCG when the follicle reaches a diameter of 17-18 mm, prior to the natural LH surge. The HCG, like LH, causes the egg to mature. Since the time of the initiation of egg maturity is precisely known, egg retrieval can be scheduled 32-38 hours later, when the egg is fully mature, yet prior to its release from the follicle. Antagonists, such as Antagon or Cetrotide, can also be used to block the LH surge when administered on a daily basis from the time that the follicle reaches 14 mm. HCG is then given to complete egg maturation when the follicle reaches 18-20 mm. Egg retrieval can then be scheduled at an optimal time.

This approach is appropriate for patients who do not produce many follicles in response to maximal stimulation protocols. It is certainly logical to use *no* medications when the same result is achieved both with and without them. This method may also appeal to patients who are opposed to the creation of extra embryos for religious reasons or those who may not be comfortable with the use of fertility-enhancing medication. This approach has the advantage of being able to be repeated on consecutive months, since the ovaries do not need a rest period to recover from the effects of the fertility medications used for controlled ovarian hyperstimulation. In addition, since the patient has only a single follicle to be aspirated, a minimal dose of Demerol can be used to manage any discomfort associated with the procedure. It is important to note that the pregnancy rate using Natural IVF is only about 6% per cycle. This approach is, for the most part, employed in only the most difficult clinical situations.

"TWEAKING" STIMULATION PROTOCOLS

Although I believe that all gonadotropins are "created equal," some physicians maintain that patients may need varying amounts of LH, as well as FSH, to produce eggs that are of maximal quality. These doctors may use LH supplementation (Luveris), in addition to pure FSH, for their IVF stimulation protocols. Some prefer to use LH containing FSH preparations, such as Menopur or Repronex, or to add HCG in minute amounts to the FSH injections. There have been many clinical comparison studies published over the past four years, but none has demonstrated a clear advantage of using LH supplementation in IVF stimulation protocols.

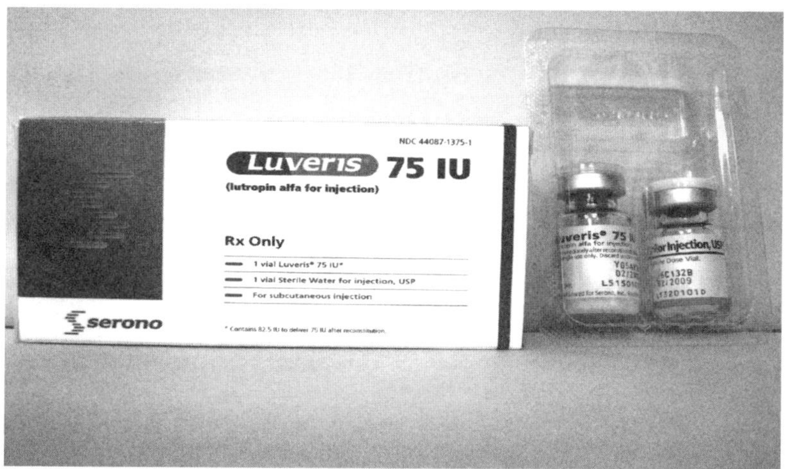

Fig. 3. ***This medication is pure LH and is used as a supplement to FSH in certain IVF protocols.***

I believe that LH supplementation may be needed only in certain cases, such as for very thin women who do not menstruate and have very low levels of FSH, LH and estradiol. These women may not respond to pure FSH, but will produce follicles when LH is added. It is important to note that the addition of LH in this situation only allows ovarian follicle development to occur; it does not necessarily ensure better egg quality in women who respond to FSH.

TRADITIONAL PROTOCOLS VS. MINIMALIST APPROACHES

Although insufficient data currently exist to allow a valid comparison between traditional IVF protocols and the "minimalist" approaches, there seems to be a growing acceptance of this new concept, which was originally developed by Dr. O. Kato, founder of one of the most prestigious IVF centers in Japan. Dr. Kato's unique approach to IVF has been successfully used in his clinics for the past 15 years, and is, I believe, one of the most intellectually courageous treatment innovations in the field of reproductive medicine. Recently, I read a translation of his book, "Infertility Without Tears," which was not only scientifically illuminating, but also poetic in its humanitarian sentiments.

Adding further credibility to Dr. Kato's approach to IVF has been the recent creation of a Society for Natural IVF, which held its first international symposium in December 2006. Apparently, an increasing number of fertility specialists are expressing interest in this approach and are using it clinically for certain patients. The minimalist approach is appealing for several reasons. It requires far fewer injections for the patient, is markedly less costly, and avoids ovarian hyperstimulation as well as the possibility of multiple births. Yet the advantage of the traditional IVF approach is that it offers multiple embryos for cryopreservation, which may ultimately result in higher pregnancy rates. It is critical that couples that are being treated for infertility are aware of this therapeutic option.

THE HIGH RESPONDER

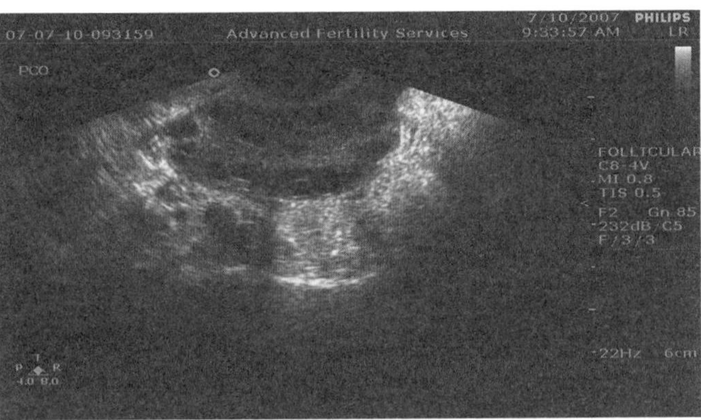

Fig. 4. ***Sonogram showing a polycystic ovary. Such patients are at high risk for ovarian hyperstimulation.***

High responders are women who produce extremely high numbers of egg follicles when stimulated with gonadotropins. These patients seldom have menstrual periods and are considered to have a form of the Polycystic Ovarian Syndrome. Their ovaries tend to contain many egg follicles, but many of the eggs contained therein are of poor quality. Relatively large proportions do not develop normally in terms of size or maturity. This results in lower pregnancy and higher miscarriage rates than would be expected.

High responders are the most difficult patients for a physician to manage. Since they are likely to produce very high levels of estrogen with small follicles, these patients run the highest risk of cycle cancellation and hospitalization for Ovarian Hyperstimulation Syndrome (OHSS). In over responders, it is important that the natural activity of the ovaries be suppressed prior to stimulation with gonadotropins and that the egg follicles be allowed to develop very slowly. This can make a big difference in the quality of the eggs produced and in the resulting pregnancy rates.

One potential drug protocol for a woman who qualifies as an over responder is to have her take birth control pills for 17 or more days in order to put the ovaries at rest. After the birth control pills have been discontinued, the woman should begin taking a daily dosage of 10 units of Lupron, to further "shut down" her ovaries. After 7-14 days of Lupron, she would start out with relatively low doses of FSH. Such patients need to be monitored more frequently than those in the other categories, as they tend to over respond very suddenly. Depending on the results of the blood tests and sonogram, an over responder's FSH dosage must be adjusted upward in small increments.

Another option for an over responder is to have her take a single injection of Depot (long-acting) Lupron on day 1 to 5 of her menstrual cycle. This will cause her ovaries to be at rest for about one month. Since it has been shown that over responders produce the best-quality eggs when their ovaries have been shut down for long periods, the injection should be repeated 30 days later. Several weeks after the second Depot Lupron injection, the woman would begin taking low doses of FSH to stimulate egg production.

POTENTIAL RISKS OF CONTROLLED OVARIAN HYPERSTIMULATION

Ovarian Hyperstimulation is a small but potentially serious, risk associated with the use of gonadotropins. In fact, all women who respond well to stimulation can be said to be hyperstimulated to some extent. However, in the Ovarian Hyperstimulation Syndrome (OHSS), an unidentified substance causes the fluid component of blood to seep through the walls of the blood vessels into the patient's abdomen and chest cavities. The dangerous result is that the blood becomes too concentrated (thick) and may be excessively prone to clotting.

Although all women who take fertility drugs experience some degree of bloating and discomfort, these symptoms are much more severe in patients with OHSS. Such patients may also experience severe abdominal distention and shortness of breath. The symptoms do not occur until 96 hours after the HCG injection

OHSS can occur when the ovaries produce higher-than-desired estrogen levels (4,000-6,000 picograms/ml) and dramatically large numbers (e.g. 40-50) of developing follicles. The most likely candidates to develop severe OHSS are those with Polycystic Ovarian Syndrome or other forms of hormonal imbalances, which result in the absence of menstrual periods. Thankfully, few women who have high levels of estrogen and large numbers of follicles develop severe OHSS. The problem, if it occurs, is usually in a mild form.

The Hyperstimulation Syndrome can be prevented if HCG is withheld for that cycle, but doing so would mean that the IVF cycle would have to be cancelled. Although the package insert for gonadotropins recommends that HCG not be administered if the patient's estrogen level exceeds 2,000 picograms/ml, most women can produce estrogen levels in the 2,000-4,000 picograms/ml range without developing problems. In clinical practice, HCG is commonly given in those circumstances. There are several strategies for dealing with excessively high levels of estrogen without canceling the IVF cycle. The simplest approach is to "coast" the patient for one or two days without medication until the estrogen level drops to a lower range before giving HCG. However, the patient must be monitored on a daily basis since the estrogen level can fall precipitously, signaling the demise of the developing eggs.

Since the hyperstimulation syndrome always resolves when a woman gets her period, the problem is self-limiting. But if a woman conceives, it can worsen dramatically—especially if she has a multiple pregnancy. Therefore, if a patient appears to be at extreme risk for OHSS, any embryos that develop can be frozen for use during a subsequent cycle. The good news is that, even if a woman develops OHSS, her risk of serious illness is low. Hospitalization is required in only about 1/800 cases, and the disorder is rarely life threatening. Only two fatalities from OHSS have been reported worldwide during the last 25 years.

THE LATE HYPERSTIMULATION SYNDROME

Late hyperstimulation occurs approximately one week after the embryo transfer. In these cases, starting at three to five days after the transfer, the woman notices that her abdomen has become markedly distended. This may indicate the onset of late hyperstimulation. The good news is that it almost always means that the woman has conceived. In fact, many pregnancies associated with late hyperstimulation are multiple gestations. Hospitalization is frequently necessary, but the problem is almost always self-limiting. Knowing that they are pregnant tends in itself to compensate for whatever treatment these women need to endure!

MONITORING

IVF patients need to be monitored to evaluate the quality and quantity of egg follicles produced. This monitoring is performed via blood hormone testing and vaginal sonograms. The results of the blood tests and sonograms need to be evaluated together to help the doctor decide how best to proceed.

Monitoring is hardly ever needed before a woman has had at least three days of stimulation. Older patients and low responders can begin their monitoring as late as the fifth day of injections. Monitoring is done on an individualized basis. In cases in which a woman has polycystic ovaries or is very thin, monitoring must be done much more frequently, even on a daily basis, since patients with polycystic ovaries are more likely to become overstimulated.

ULTRASOUND

Vaginal ultrasound enables the doctor to evaluate the number and size of the follicles the patient is producing. Egg follicle size is the most important criterion for determining the optimal time for egg retrieval. Mature eggs can be expected to be found in follicles having a diameter of 16-22 mm. Once the majority of the developing follicles have reached this size, HCG can be taken and the retrieval can be planned.

BLOOD HORMONE LEVELS

The hormones that need to be monitored for IVF cycles are estrogen, LH (Luteinizing Hormone) and progesterone. Each gives important information as to the patient's response to stimulation.

Estrogen

A woman's blood estrogen level, which is the second most important criterion for timing the patient's egg retrieval, increases as the number and size of her developing egg follicles increase. Both the number and development of the follicles contribute to the level of estrogen. For example, if a woman has 5 to 6 developing follicles measuring 18-20 mm, and her estrogen level is measured at 1,200 pg/ml, that level may signal that the follicles have reached maturity and that she is ready for her HCG injection. However, if that same level of estrogen were seen in a woman with many follicles measuring only 10-12 mm each, it would mean that she was over responding to the medication and that her dosage needed to be drastically reduced or discontinued.

Luteinizing Hormone (LH)
The measurement of Luteinizing Hormone is very important, since its elevation indicates that the body has initiated the final step of egg maturation and that the follicles will rupture and release the eggs in 36-42 hours. When patients are using Lupron, LH production is prevented 99% of the time, so there is no real concern for premature release of the eggs prior to retrieval. However, when non-Lupron protocols are used (Pure Gonadotropin Protocol, European Protocol), LH levels must be monitored to anticipate premature egg release. The inclusion of LH antagonists in non-Lupron regimens can prevent premature egg release.

Progesterone
Monitoring progesterone levels is useful in determining whether there will be a potential problem with embryo implantation. A rise in progesterone levels, which occurs as a result of the natural LH surge or an HCG injection, causes the lining of the uterus to be prepared for potential implantation by an embryo.

Occasionally, a woman's progesterone level will increase prematurely to a level of more than 4.0 mg/ml prior to administration of the HCG. This may be of no clinical consequence or it may mean that her uterine lining is not well synchronized with the other elements of her cycle. If the endometrial lining does not have a normal appearance on an ultrasound examination, the woman can proceed with the retrieval but her embryos should be frozen for use during a later cycle.

SUMMARY

A variety of fertility drugs can be administered to stimulate patients to produce multiple egg follicles in the initial phase of an IVF treatment cycle. These drugs are prescribed in a highly individualized manner for each patient, using different combinations at varying dosages. Treatment protocols are based on a patient's unique clinical characteristics as well as their previous responses to ovarian stimulation. Regular monitoring via ultrasound and blood hormone testing is necessary to produce a group of uniformly mature oocytes, while at the same time preventing the occurrence of the ovarian hyperstimulation syndrome.

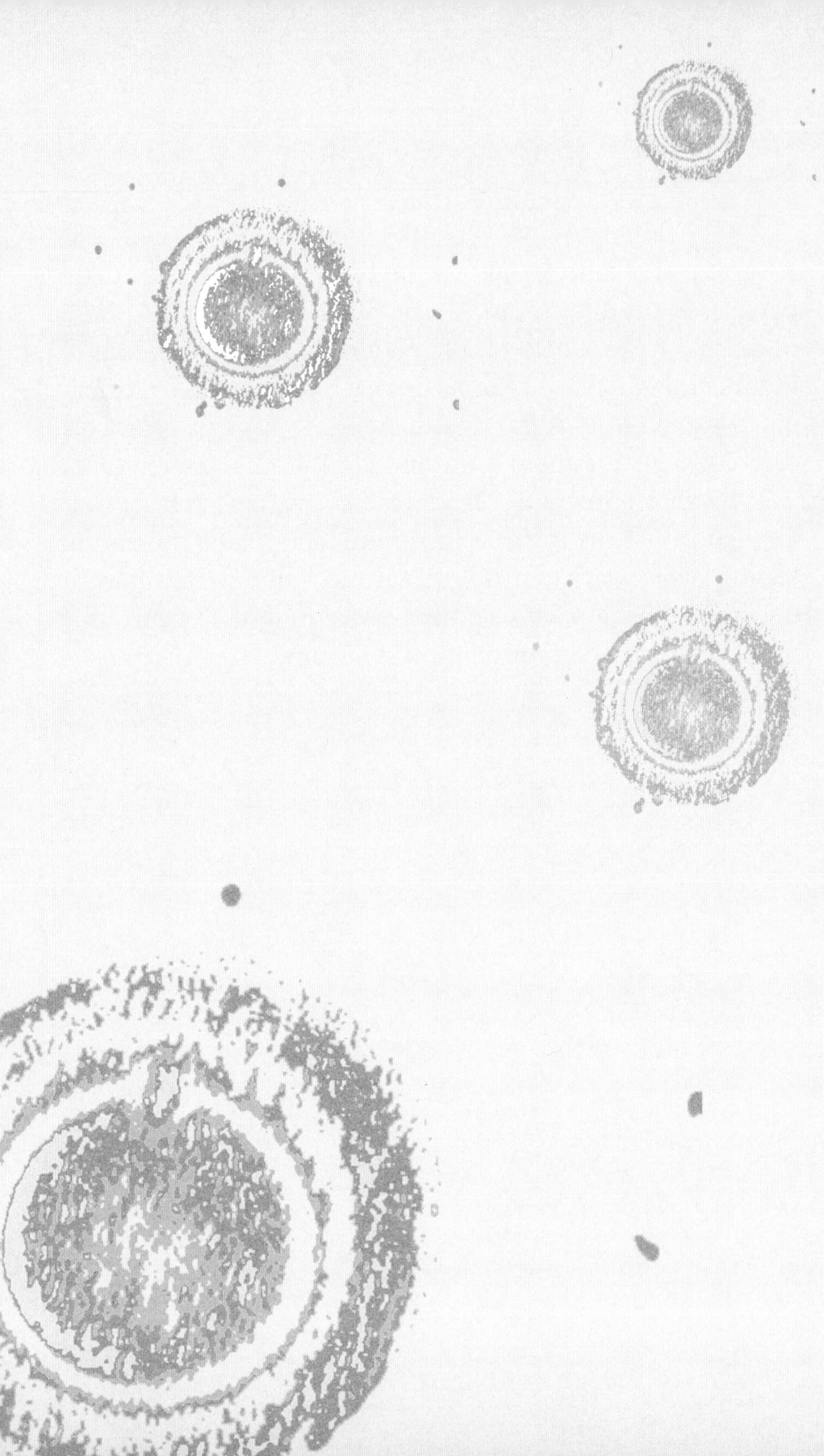

CHAPTER 8

IN VITRO FERTILIZATION: *THE EGG RETRIEVAL*

The part of *In Vitro* Fertilization (IVF) that concerns prospective patients the most is the procedure to remove eggs from their ovaries. However, in my experience, the vast majority of women who have undergone an egg retrieval procedure agree that it was not nearly as painful or traumatic as they had anticipated. It is very normal, as well as wise, to fear undergoing any medical procedure. No matter how minor a procedure is said to be, all have some degree of discomfort and risk. The good news is that the egg retrieval procedure is minimally invasive and has an excellent track record with respect to safety. To put everything into perspective, compared with childbirth, the egg retrieval process is much shorter and certainly less painful.

Prior to 1986, in the early days of IVF, the only way to retrieve eggs was via laparoscopy—a surgical procedure that required general anesthesia, took between one and two hours to perform, and left the woman with incisions to heal, stitches to remove and a significant degree of discomfort for days afterward. All that has now changed, and a patient's eggs are removed via a small ultrasound-guided needle placed through the wall of the vagina and into the ovary. The procedure is extremely safe, causes minimal discomfort, and rarely takes more than ten minutes to perform. The drawing in the figure below shows the anatomic relationships between the female reproductive organs that permit the nonsurgical approach for the removal of eggs from the ovaries.

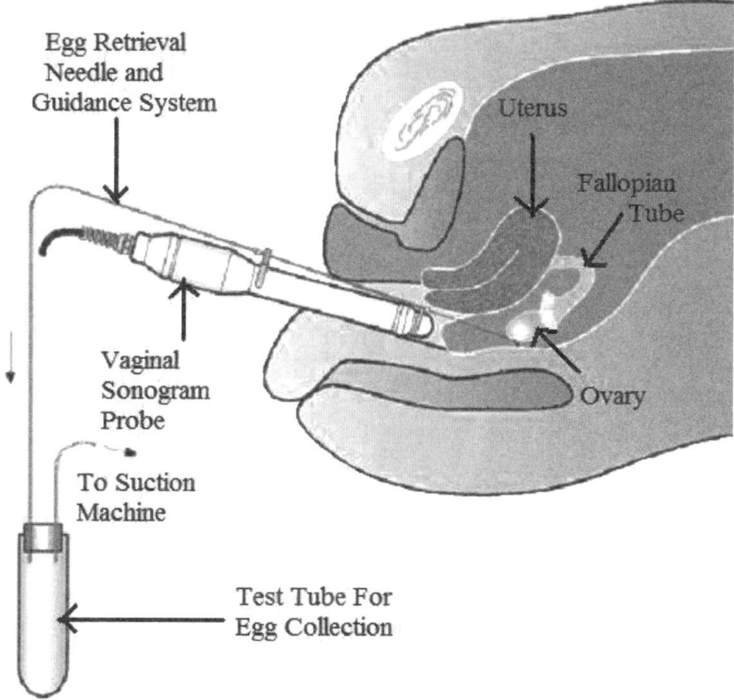

Fig. 1. ***Schematic drawing of the egg retrieval procedure.***

BEFORE THE RETRIEVAL

The most important thing to know is that you must not eat or drink after midnight prior to egg retrieval. This is an important safety precaution that should be observed, even though the anesthetic used for the retrieval is not as strong as that used for major surgery. A general "rule of thumb" is that the stomach should always be empty at least six hours prior to any medical procedure in order to prevent a rare but serious complication called aspiration pneumonia.

If you are anxious about the procedure, which is normal for "first-timers," discuss what frightens or concerns you with your doctor. Just sharing your concerns with someone goes a long way in helping dispel all fears. If you anticipate having difficulty sleeping the night before the retrieval, taking Tylenol-PM or 25 mg of the allergy drug Benadryl will be helpful as a sleep aid. Should you become extremely thirsty, sucking on an ice cube is permissible. If you are prone to having the "shakes" from low blood sugar, briefly sucking on a piece of hard candy is safe. For diabetic patients, it will be necessary to modify the morning insulin dosage, depending on the time of the egg retrieval. This should be discussed with your physician.

The male partner should abstain from sexual activity for one to two days prior to the retrieval to guarantee an adequate sperm specimen.

RETRIEVAL DAY PREPARATION

When a patient arrives for her egg retrieval, she will be escorted to the treatment area where she will meet with the anesthesiologist and have pre-procedure counseling. The patient will then don an examining gown and empty her bladder. She will subsequently lie down on the exam table and be positioned in the same way as for routine sonograms or gynecological exams. Then she will be connected to monitoring equipment that will continuously record the heart rate, blood pressure and blood oxygen content throughout the procedure. An anesthesiologist will start an intravenous line for the administration of an anesthetic agent called Propofol. This agent induces a peaceful sleeping state, during which the patient will feel no pain and will have no recollection of the procedure having been performed. Upon awakening, the patient will not feel the nausea or extreme dizziness associated with traditional anesthetics. Rather, she will awake feeling as if she had a refreshing nap, but will want to go back to sleep for a while longer. Having received this anesthetic myself for the removal of a kidney stone, I can attest to the fact that with Propofol there is no pain, no memories, as well as no nausea, vomiting or "hangover" that is typically experienced with other anesthetic agents. It is also very safe, since it does not stop your breathing nor does it require assisted ventilation. Moreover, there is no risk for aspiration of gastric contents or other secretions into the lungs.

THE PROCEDURE

During the retrieval, the sonographer, doctor and a nurse work together as a team in order to harvest the eggs. While the patient is asleep, the sonographer inserts a vaginal probe and visualizes the patient's ovaries. The probe has a needle guide attached to it, which is aligned to follow a computer-generated path into an ovarian egg follicle. Using the needle guidance system, the doctor inserts a retrieval needle through the wall of the vagina into each ovary under direct visual control on a video monitor. The contents of each egg follicle are suctioned into a test tube. Generally, all the eggs in an ovary can be recovered with a single puncture, so the procedure is usually accomplished with one needle puncture per side.

A clear yellow fluid will emerge from the follicle, which hopefully contains a mature egg. The egg itself is microscopic, so it cannot be seen to be floating in the follicular fluid. Using a specialized microscope, the egg is located in the follicular fluid by the embryologist, who quickly transfers it into a special liquid "broth", called tissue culture media, and places it in an incubator.

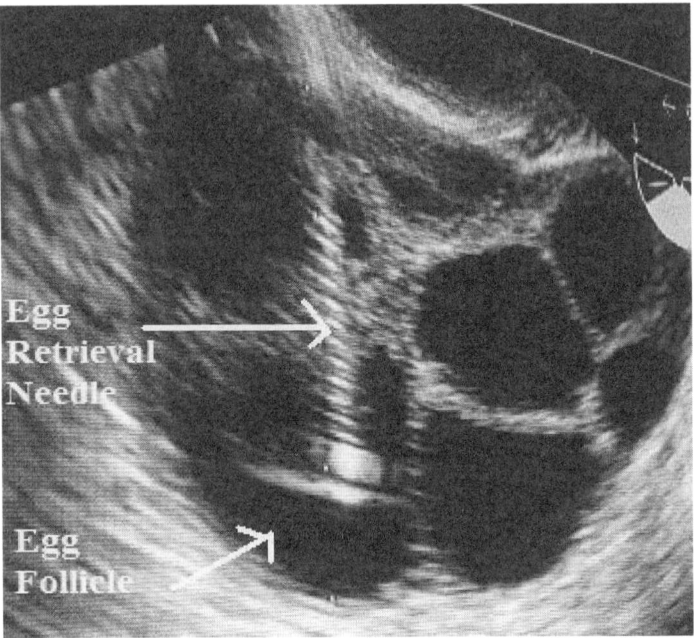

Fig. 2. ***Sonographic view as egg retrieval procedure is actually being performed by the physician.***

After the Retrieval

The patient usually rests for one to two hours after the retrieval, after which she is able to go home. By law, anyone having anesthesia is not permitted to drive a car or use potentially dangerous equipment for the next 24 hours. This is because coordination and reflexes may be impaired after general anesthesia, as some of the drugs used may have a lingering effect in the body. Fortunately, Propofol is cleared from the system rapidly, so patients recover relatively quickly. Nevertheless, although the patient may feel "normal" very soon after the procedure, she should observe the law and exercise extra caution in all activities for the next 24 hours. Some patients experience abdominal cramping and dizziness after the procedure, but these have usually subsided once they are ready to leave the recovery area. Vaginal bleeding from the puncture sites is common. It is much lighter than a period and will subside after 48 hours.

Although there is an extremely low complication rate from the retrieval process, any time a needle is passed into the human body there is the potential for infection or internal bleeding. Infections can develop either through bacterial contamination from the vagina or from multiple inadvertent punctures of the intestines. The retrieval needles are very fine, so a single intestinal puncture seals up immediately without bacterial contamination and infection. Likewise, bleeding into the abdomen rarely occurs. When it does happen, it is usually the result of the puncture of an ovarian vein or artery. Bleeding may also happen when a patient takes too much aspirin or non-steroidal anti-inflammatory drugs, like Motrin or Aleve. Other complications include torsion (twisting) of the ovary and bleeding into an already aspirated follicle cyst. Bleeding into the urinary bladder, resulting in blood-tinged urine after the retrieval, is common and is no cause for alarm as long as the urine is not bright red and there is no difficulty with urination.

The majority of serious complications other than infection are usually recognized prior to a patient's discharge from the IVF facility. If a complication is suspected, a patient will be sent to a back-up hospital facility for observation and treatment. The treatment of complications is a coordinated effort between the appropriate hospital specialists and the IVF doctor. In the time interval between the egg retrieval and the transfer, if the patient experiences symptoms such as a fever greater than 101.5F, with chills and increasing abdominal pain, the IVF center should be notified so that the symptoms can be evaluated and treatment given. If a patient lives far from the IVF center, she should go to the closest hospital emergency room. It is crucial that the treating physician be in contact with the IVF doctor in order to facilitate both diagnosis and treatment.

SUMMARY

Although it is natural to experience a great deal of anxiety at the prospect of having eggs removed from your ovaries, you can rest assured that little discomfort will be experienced both during and after the procedure. Furthermore, the procedure has an excellent safety record. The chances of a patient having a major complication from oocyte retrieval are low. The relative ease of the egg retrieval procedure enables patients who require multiple attempts at IVF to persevere with their treatments in order to maximize their chances for pregnancy.

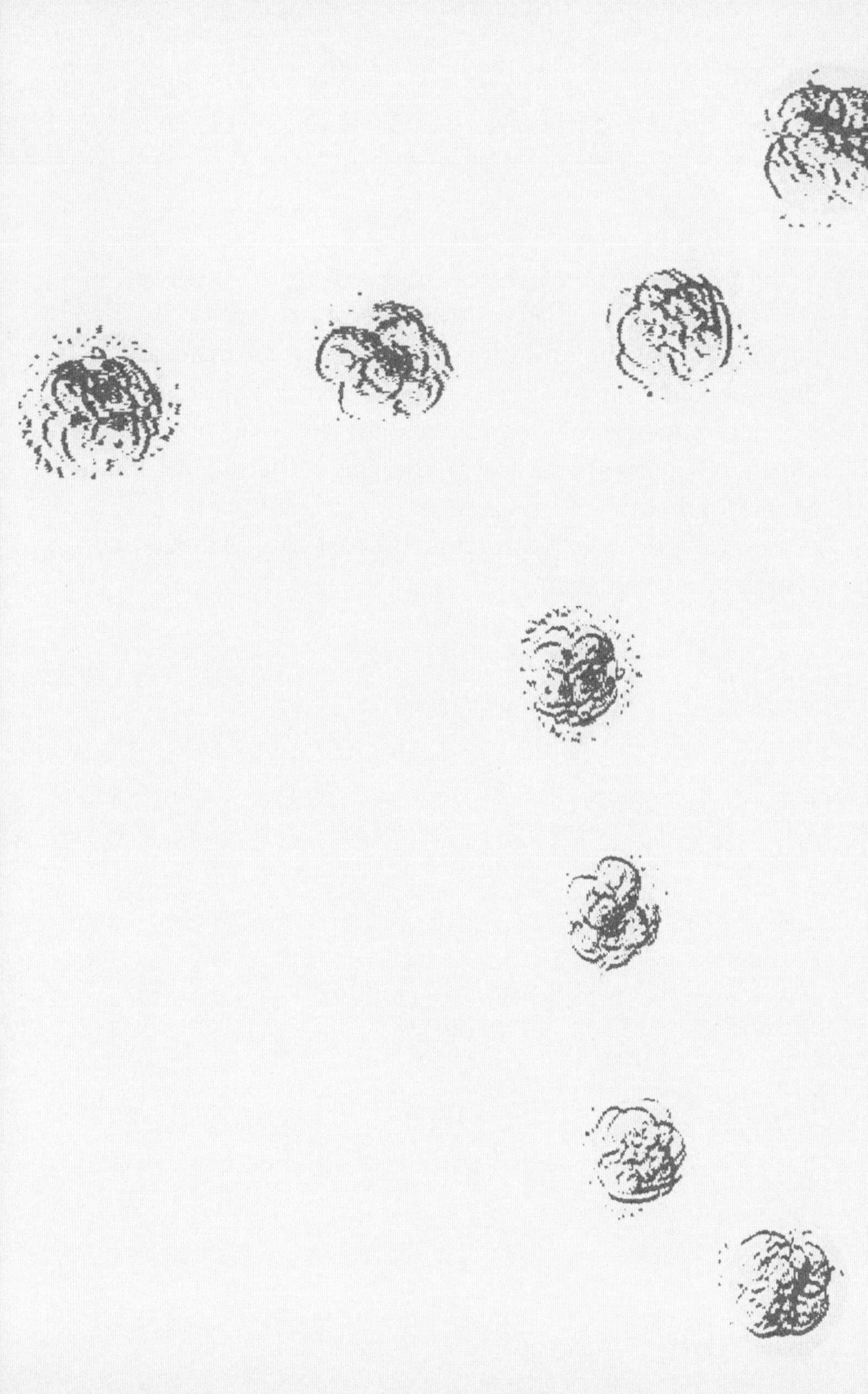

CHAPTER 9

THE MALE COMPONENT IN IVF

Thus far, we have focused almost exclusively on the production of mature eggs. But unless you possess the secret of cloning, it is obviously impossible to make a baby without sperm. The good news is that it is no longer necessary for the male to produce millions, thousands, or even hundreds of sperm in order for conception to take place. With today's technology, pregnancy is possible even if there is just one live sperm available to unite with a single mature egg.

THE SPERM SPECIMEN

Compared with a woman, who needs to undergo an oocyte retrieval for *In Vitro* Fertilization (IVF), the man usually has a relatively easy time of it. He needs only to produce a sperm specimen to be used to fertilize the retrieved eggs. Some time after the retrieval, the male will be asked to ejaculate into a sterile specimen container, which he will then give directly to the embryologist and/or andrologist. (Don't worry—a private room with some erotic books and movies is provided!) The sperm is then "processed" and separated from the seminal fluid via one of several different techniques and is subsequently used for natural insemination or assisted Intracytoplasmic Sperm Injection (ICSI) of the eggs retrieved from his partner's ovaries.

Although it may seem simple enough for a man to produce a sperm specimen on demand, many men may have difficulties in doing so. There is always the possibility that the psychological pressures of a "command performance" may render any male incapable of ejaculation. The potential catastrophe of temporary impotence on the day of egg retrieval can easily be avoided by the cryopreservation (freezing) of a semen sample prior to the day of the egg retrieval. If a man is unable to produce sperm for fertilization in a timely fashion, his cryopreserved semen is readily available for fertilizing his wife's oocytes.

Unfortunately, there are the occasional instances when a man will not heed the recommendation for a frozen back-up sperm sample. Such a situation recently occurred in my practice. After his wife's egg retrieval, which yielded 15 mature oocytes, Alan, a 38-year-old attorney, could not produce a sperm specimen. At first he was embarrassed at his inability to perform; shortly thereafter, he became distraught to the point that I sensed he was close to an emotional meltdown. To make matters worse, his wife—fearful that the IVF cycle was doomed because of her husband's problem—became very anxious and put more pressure on Alan to ejaculate. Her response only made matters worse. In order to avoid a total disaster, the couple needed emergency counseling and a little blue pill called Viagra for Alan. After a brief discussion about how stress and anxiety inhibit a man's ability to maintain an erection and ejaculate, the couple was advised to go out for a nice lunch, complemented by a bottle of wine. They were specifically advised not to discuss anything pertaining to their IVF experience, but rather to concentrate on having a romantic "date." Two hours later, they returned to the office, relaxed and a bit tipsy. They headed directly to a private room, from which they emerged ten minutes later with the sperm specimen.

If nothing can be done to produce a sperm specimen on the day of egg retrieval, it is possible to freeze the eggs in the unfertilized state. These eggs can then be fertilized at a later date and subsequently transferred. While this option may appear to be a reasonable one, it is less likely to result in a viable pregnancy.

WHEN THE SPERM COUNT IS ZERO ...

Some men may have no sperm in their ejaculate (azospermia). This can result from blockages in the epididymal ducts that lead from the testes to the outside world. Such blockages can be a result of infection or from having been born without such ducts, which is called a congenital absence. Although the conditions vary in causation, they are identical in that the testes produce normal amounts of sperm but the sperm are unable to exit the male reproductive tract. In these cases, hormonal testing can demonstrate that there is, in fact, sperm contained inside the testicles. Just as in the case of the female, where low levels of FSH and LH suggest the presence of eggs in the ovaries, low levels of FSH and LH indicate the probable presence of sperm in the testes.

Yet high levels of these hormones in both sexes indicate that there is no sperm or that there are no eggs present in the gonadal tissues. Such hormonal testing usually eliminates the need for surgical biopsy of the testes to diagnose cases of absolute male sterility.

Prior to the early 1990s, there was no technology available to treat these conditions, and all azospermic men were condemned to a lifetime of absolute sterility. Fortunately, two techniques are now readily available to extract sperm directly from the testicles: Microsurgical Epididymal Sperm Aspiration (MESA) and Testicular Sperm Extraction (TESE). With these techniques, sufficient numbers of viable sperm may be obtained to fertilize oocytes, employing the direct injection (ICSI) of a single sperm into each egg obtained by

IVF. Thus, fatherhood may still be a possibility even when the sperm count is zero.

MICROEPIDIDYMAL SPERM ASPIRATION (MESA)

MESA is used to extract sperm from men with an obvious blockage in their epididymal ducts. This is frequently the case when a man has had a vasectomy or a failed vasectomy reversal. It is a nonsurgical procedure, which is performed with a local anesthetic while the patient is under conscious sedation (Demerol and Versed) or asleep after an injection of Propofol. A urologist will locate an area immediately before the site of the obstruction of the epididymal tube, which is in the top portion of the scrotal sac. This area is similar to a dam that contains an accumulation of live and dead sperm. Using a highly developed sense of touch, the urologist enters the area with a very fine needle in order to remove a specimen, which is a tiny droplet of fluid containing viable sperm. The sperm obtained in this manner are not active swimmers like those found in an ejaculated specimen. Rather, live sperm are identified by their twitching tails. Because of their relatively low numbers and poor motility, sperm obtained in this manner are inadequate for intrauterine insemination. Rather, the sperm must be injected directly into eggs obtained by IVF. MESA is performed on the same day as the egg retrieval or in the 24-hour period preceding it. Excess viable sperm can sometimes be cryopreserved for subsequent use in another IVF attempt.

TESTICULAR SPERM EXTRACTION (TESE)

TESE is a more frequently performed sperm extraction

procedure than is MESA. It is used in instances in which no sperm can be obtained with MESA and in cases where azospermia is not due to an obvious sperm duct blockage. The procedure is performed on the same day as—or on the day prior to—the egg retrieval. The male is either under conscious sedation with the testes numbed with a local anesthetic or—preferably—put to sleep with Propofol. Using a specialized biopsy needle, the urologist extracts tiny pieces of testicular tissue from multiple sites in the testes. The embryologist then conducts a microscopic examination of the testicular tissue obtained, searching for areas of sperm-containing tissue. This part of the procedure is painstakingly time consuming, since finding sperm in this type of tissue is about as difficult as finding the proverbial "needle in a haystack." It is not unusual for an embryologist to spend three to five hours attempting to find enough sperm to be injected into the eggs retrieved from his partner's ovaries. Although sperm harvested via TESE yield similar fertilization rates as MESA, the sperm from the testes are more difficult for the embryologist to work with since they exhibit even less movement than do those obtained by MESA.

The unfortunate reality is that MESA and TESE procedures do not always yield sperm. Even with multiple tissue samples obtained by an experienced urologist, an embryologist may not find viable sperm after hours of searching under the microscope. When this happens, it is obviously devastating to the couple. I always discuss this dismal possibility with prospective patients well in advance of the procedure. In addition, I give them the option of ordering a donor sperm specimen as a back-up scenario, in the case that sperm are not obtained. Many couples decide to avail themselves of this option in order to maximize their chances for a successful outcome.

Patients are usually able to return home two hours after the procedure. Since an anesthetic is used, patients should not drive a car or use power tools for 24 hours after the procedure due to residual effects of sedation. Couples need to make arrangements to have a driver take them home, since their reflexes will be impaired after anesthesia; in fact, it is illegal to drive for the prescribed period of time after these procedures.

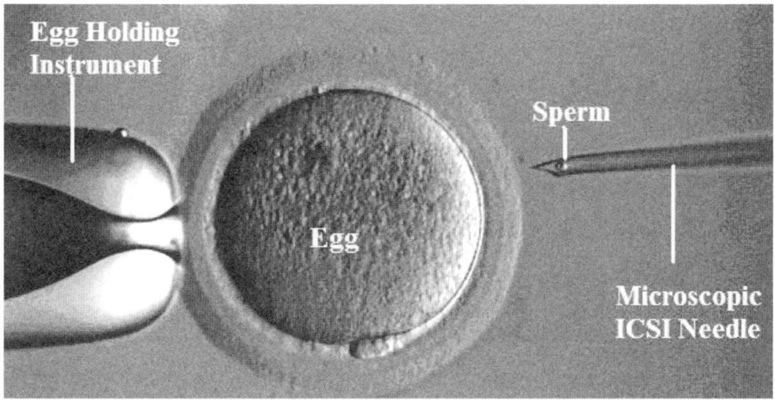

Fig. 1. ***A Microscopic view of ICSI as the embryologist injects a single sperm into the egg.***

MESA AND TESE SUCCESS RATES

Both MESA and TESE make the successful outcome of an IVF cycle even more difficult, since another variable—obtaining viable sperm—has been added. Although sperm obtained via MESA and TESE yield good fertilization rates with ICSI (50-80%), pregnancy rates cannot be expected to be equally high. The key to predicting the chances for a successful outcome with MESA/TESE is the age of the female partner, her ability to produce many ooctyes and any history of previous pregnancies. If a woman is 38- to 40-years-old and produces only 3 to 4 oocytes in response to fertility drugs, chances for a successful outcome are unlikely and this treatment option is not advised. If, however, the female partner is young and produces many oocytes, pregnancy rates are similar to those resulting from regular IVF.

When a testicular biopsy is recommended to evaluate azoospermia, couples should be aware of the possibility of combining the biopsy with the IVF retrieval. A portion of the testicular specimen can be used to look for sperm to fertilize his partner's eggs. The remainder will be sent to a laboratory for pathological examination. This will give the couple a chance for a pregnancy at the same time that the diagnostic procedure is being performed.

SUMMARY

With the development of ICSI, IVF technology has become the "gold standard" treatment for all types of male infertility. When a male has a low sperm count, poor motility or abnormal morphology (shape), ICSI can facilitate the entrance of a single sperm into an egg so that the process of fertilization can commence in cases in which it would otherwise be impossible. The true miracle is when a man who produces no sperm is able to father his own biological child with TESE/MESA and IVF.

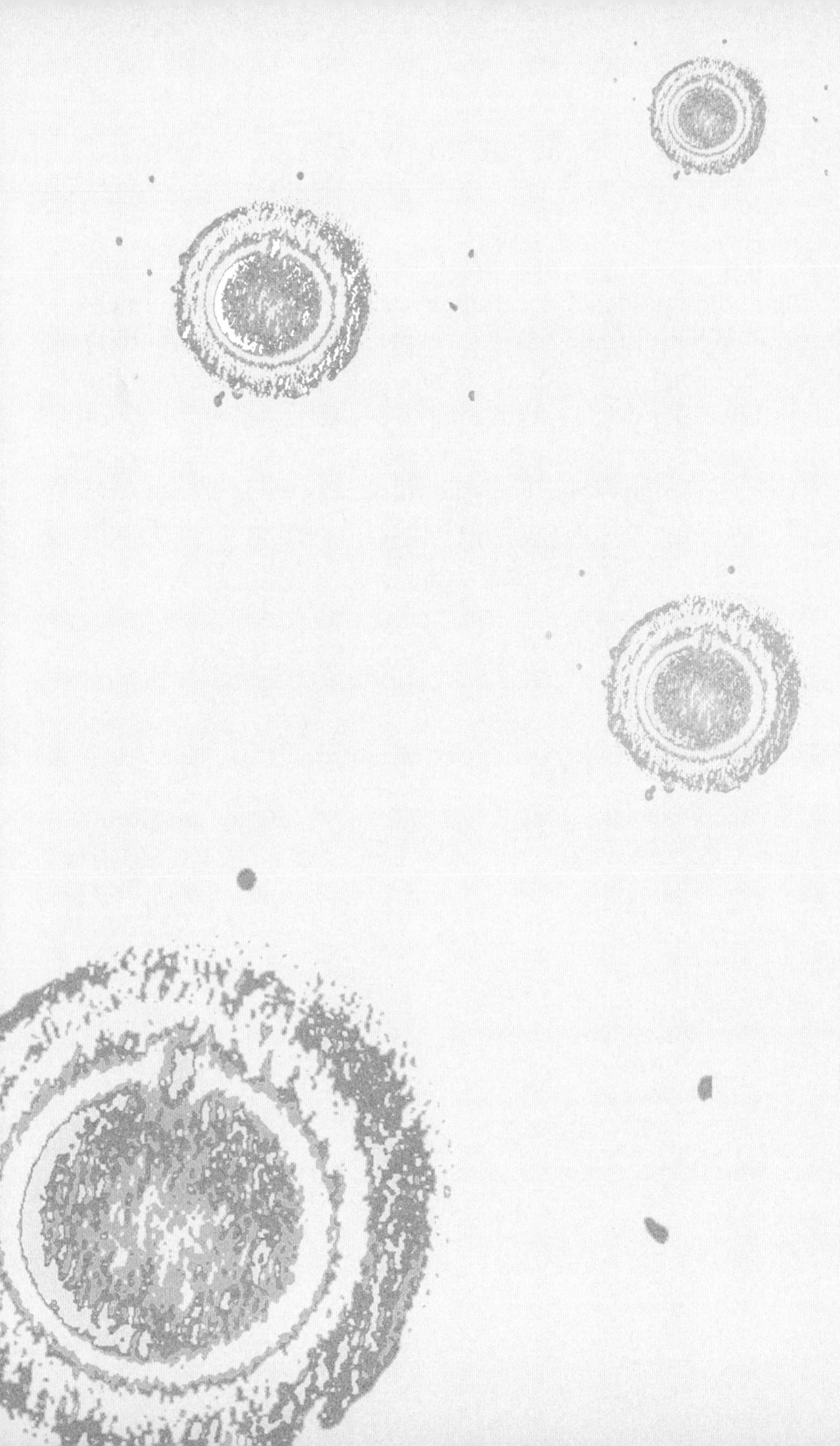

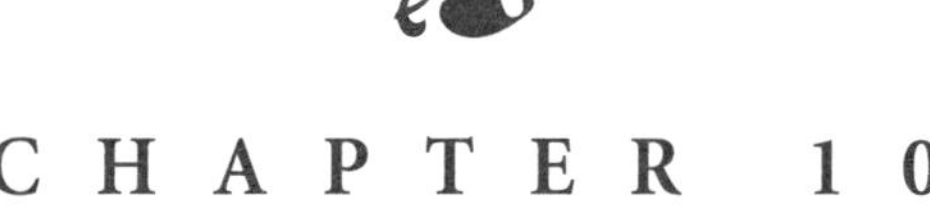

CHAPTER 10

THE IVF LABORATORY:

Fertilization, Embryo Transfer and Cryopreservation

The three most important elements for maximizing the chances for the successful fertilization of oocytes are the skill of the embryologist, the caliber of the IVF lab, and the quality and maturity of the eggs.

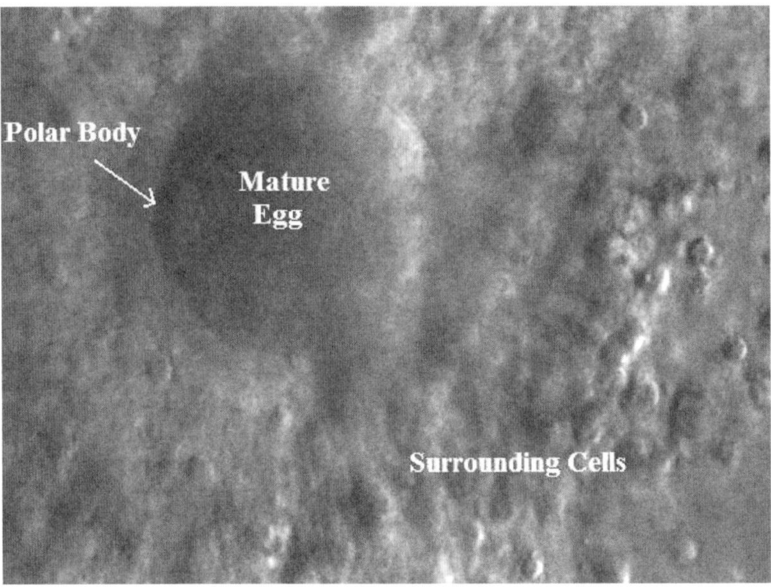

Fig. 1. ***An egg in follicular fluid located by the embryologist under a microscope.***

THE EMBRYOLOGIST

A clinical embryologist is a laboratory scientist who, in addition to being an expert in all aspects of reproduction on the cellular and genetic levels, has been extensively trained in techniques for growing and maintaining cells in tissue culture systems. Since the embryologist maintains full responsibility for the IVF laboratory, he or she must be meticulous in adhering to high standards of technique and quality control, since human eggs and embryos are incredibly sensitive to their environmental conditions. The major clinical functions performed by the embryologist in the IVF lab are:

1. Locating the eggs within the follicular fluid that is removed from patients' ovaries
2. Grading the eggs in terms of maturity
3. Maintaining media and culture conditions that will allow the cells to grow for the required period of time
4. Preparing sperm for natural insemination or Intracytoplasmic Sperm Injection (ICSI)
5. Performing micromanipulation (ICSI, Assisted Hatching, Embryo Biopsy for PGD)

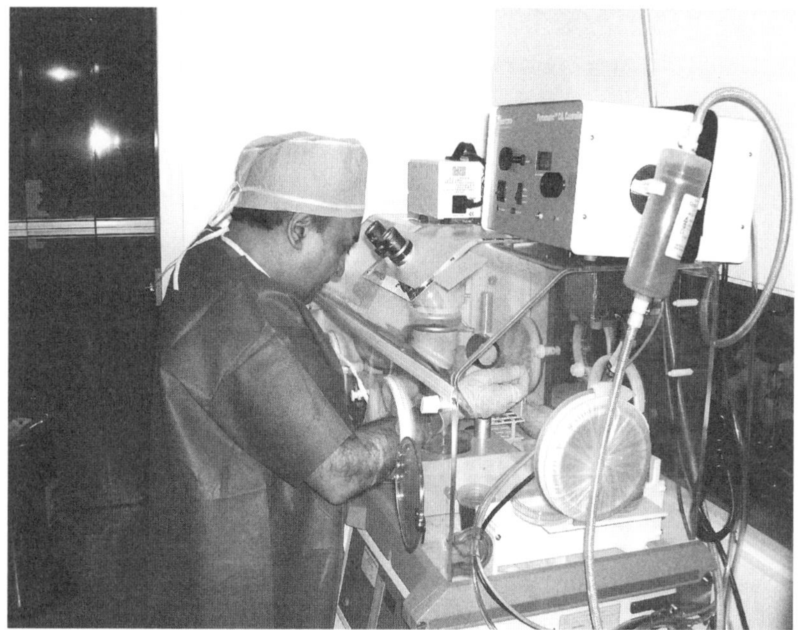

Fig. 2. ***An embryologist locating eggs in follicular fluid that has been removed during an egg retrieval.***

Since fertilization rates depend on egg quality, a critical responsibility of the embryologist is to evaluate the newly retrieved eggs in terms of maturity and structural integrity. The embryologist can gauge the maturity of an egg by examining the crown of cells that surround it (the corona radiata). If these surrounding cells appear expanded or enlarged and have a specific, recognizable look, the egg can be assumed to have reached Metaphase II and be ready for fertilization. If the eggs appear immature, however, they will be maintained in the incubator and fertilization will be delayed until the oocytes reach the Metaphase II stage.

If a couple's fertilization rate turns out to be much poorer than expected, it may mean either that the eggs were less mature than could be predicted by their outward appearance or that they were mature, but of poor genetic quality.

It was once believed that stripping immature eggs of their surrounding cells would assist the fertilization process by making it easier for the sperm to reach the eggs. We now know that this practice interferes with nature and can actually impede fertilization—except when the sperm needs to be injected directly inside the egg. In the process of natural fertilization, the cumulus cells surrounding the egg produce not only hormones, but also many complex biochemical factors that regulate egg growth, development and, ultimately, fertilization.

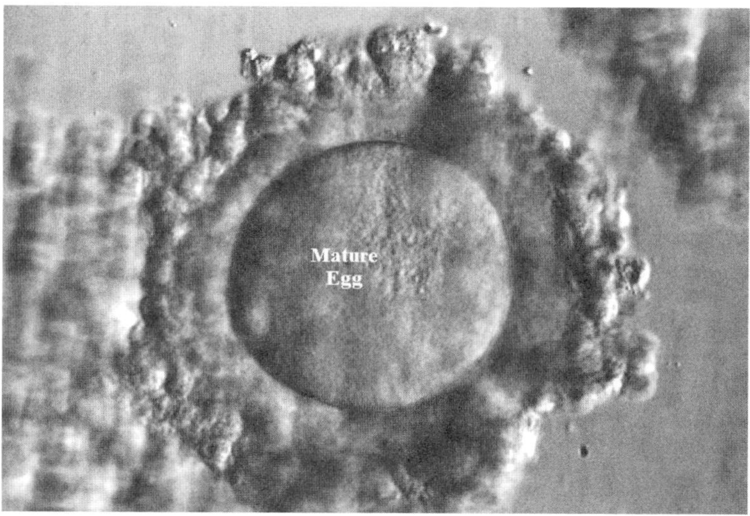

Fig. 3. ***This is a mature egg that is being prepared for ICSI by removing the surrounding cells.***

THE IVF LABORATORY

The best way to evaluate the quality of an IVF laboratory is through its fertilization and embryonic growth rates. Actual live birth rates do not accurately reflect an IVF lab's proficiency, since those rates depend on the patients that are treated. Obviously, a clinic that treats patients with a lower statistical chance of conception (e.g. older patients; patients with endometriosis, polycystic ovaries, unexplained infertility, multiple IVF failures, unexplained infertility) will have a lower clinical "live birth rate" than an IVF center whose patient population is younger and primarily affected by tubal and male factors. Although the pregnancy rates of two such clinics would be quite different, the fertilization and embryo growth rates of their IVF labs could be the same.

As IVF physicians, we are continuously evaluating our laboratory's performance since that aspect of the treatment is so critical for the possibility of obtaining a pregnancy. We evaluate the lab objectively on the basis of its functions: to fertilize eggs and to grow embryos. From a laboratory quality control perspective, if the eggs obtained are mature, the fertilization rates should be at least 60%. Although embryo growth rates largely depend on egg quality, some eggs from most patients should be able to grow and develop to the 6-8-cell stage after three days in the incubator. In addition, the ability of some eggs to reach the blastocyst stage (thousands of cells) after 5 days in culture is a further confirmation that the conditions in the laboratory are satisfactory.

In order to maintain a successful IVF program, there must be a constant, on-going evaluation process conducted by the embryologist and the doctor. The embryologist always discusses the quality of the eggs that a patient produces during a treatment cycle with the clinician. This gives the physician important insight into the need for future fine-tuning of the ovarian stimulation protocols. Likewise, if a decline in fertilization or embryo growth rates is observed, the embryologist must isolate and correct its cause. For example, an embryologist may notice that the fertilization rate is lower and the growth rate slower for embryos grown in a certain incubator compared with those grown in the other incubators in the lab. He or she will then not use that particular incubator until it is recalibrated and reevaluated by demonstrating that mouse eggs are able to fertilize and grow in it. Only after such stringent quality control will the incubator be used to grow patients' embryos.

The bottom line is that the quality of an IVF program and its laboratory is generally an all-or-nothing proposition; that is, a program that is not properly managed will produce zero pregnancies, because it is extremely difficult to fertilize human eggs or grow human embryos in a laboratory that is not well run. All lab conditions must be perfect in order to even keep embryos alive to the point of transfer. Should the laboratory be less than perfect, there will no embryos to transfer and the lab will be unable to produce a single pregnancy. A well-run lab, on the other hand, may produce either many or few pregnancies, depending on the age of the female patients and other patient selection criteria.

I believe that all the IVF programs that are currently members of the Society of Assisted Reproductive Technology (S.A.R.T.) are legitimate and have acceptable pregnancy rates. Be aware, too, that IVF labs are closely inspected and monitored for quality control issues by government agencies, such as the State Department of Health, the Center for Disease Control (CDC) and the Food and Drug Administration (FDA).

Today, the techniques, equipment and culture media used to fertilize eggs and grow embryos are quite standardized. Virtually all labs grow their embryos in fluid culture media that have been commercially produced using strict standards of quality control. This is a vast difference from the early days of IVF, when each lab had to produce its own media—the quality of which was easily compromised based on impurities or an unfavorable mineral content in the water that was the basis for the media. Most IVF labs today also use similar types of incubators to house their developing embryos. The incubators need to be carefully monitored so that the carbon dioxide content and pH remain in the proper range, since any change in the acid/base balance of the media can adversely affect embryonic growth. In fact, virtually all of today's embryos are cultured in a medium that is covered with a very thin layer of mineral oil, which serves both to ensure strict control of the pH and to shield the embryo from any possibility of potential contamination.

CO-CULTURE

The concept of co-culture, which was in vogue about ten years ago, calls for the addition of living cells to the commercially produced media that are normally used to maintain the eggs, sperm and developing embryos. The theory is that the addition of living cells from the reproductive tract of the patient, another woman, or animal will secrete critical—but yet unknown—substances that will aid in embryo growth and development. Co-culture is rarely used, except in rare instances in which a couple's embryos do not develop normally in standard culture media. If co-culture cells are used, they should come from the patient's own body since the use of human or cow cells could be a source of viral or prion (the agent causing Mad Cow Disease) contamination of the embryos. In fact, the Center for Disease Control and the Federal Drug Administration do not allow the use of blood products or cells derived from other individuals or animals in IVF culture systems. Co-culture cells may originate from the patient's own uterine lining (endometrium) cells or the cumulus cells that are removed with the oocyte at time of retrieval.

THE PROCESS OF FERTILIZATION

After the retrieval, the eggs are placed in Petri dishes filled with tissue culture media, which is essentially a complex nutrient broth that contains a large number of natural substances created to support embryo growth and development.

Several hours need to elapse after the retrieval, in order to allow the eggs to adjust to their new environment prior to starting the process of their fertilization.

After evaluating the maturity of each egg, the embryologist segregates the mature ones and adds 25,000-50,000 of the most active sperm in proximity to each egg. Then "Mother Nature" performs her magic, allowing a single sperm to penetrate the zona pellucida (outer shell) of each egg, while excluding all others. Any eggs deemed to be immature are allowed to remain in the culture medium for several more hours, since some eggs are capable of completing their maturation in the laboratory. Late maturing eggs can then be fertilized.

If the embryologist has noticed that after being processed, the sperm are moving at too low a velocity to make natural penetration of the egg likely (in our laboratory, less than 60 microns/second), fertilization can be facilitated by the injection of a single sperm directly into each egg. This procedure is called Intracytoplasmic Sperm Injection (ICSI).

INTRACYTOPLASMIC SPERM INJECTION

Perhaps the most exciting scientific breakthrough to occur in reproductive medicine in the 20th century was the development of ICSI. ICSI has truly revolutionized the process of infertility treatment by making it possible for men with poor sperm counts and barely twitching motility to fertilize their partners' eggs with approximately the same success rates (60%) as men with normal sperm counts.

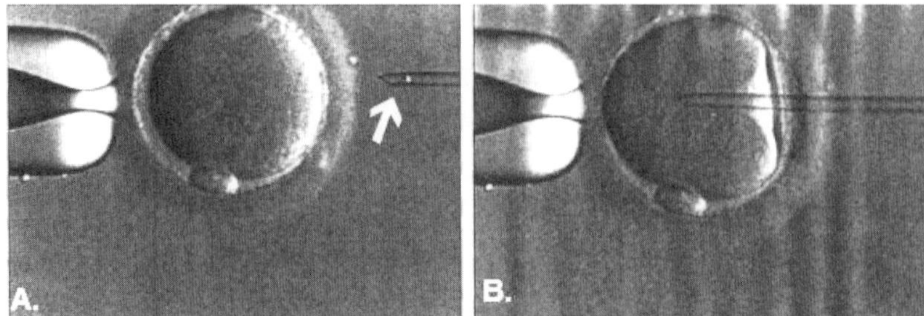

Fig. 4. A. ***ICSI: While the egg is held in place by a microscopic suction instrument, a sperm, contained in the needle, is ready to be injected into the egg.***
B. ICSI-2: The sperm injection.

ICSI is an extremely delicate microscopic robotic technique that demands great skill on the part of the embryologist. The target—the egg—measures only 1/100 of the size of a pinhead, and the sperm is a mere 1/400 of the size of the egg.

Before ICSI can be performed, the embryologist must strip the eggs of their surrounding cells. This permits a detailed evaluation of the eggs' state of maturity. If they have not yet reached maturity at Metaphase II, the procedure must be delayed for several hours until they reach that stage. Not all eggs reach maturity; those that do not reach maturity cannot be fertilized.

To perform ICSI, the embryologist places the active sperm in an immobilizing fluid medium. Then, using a very fine needle, the tail of the sperm is crushed to render it incapable of movement. The incapacitated sperm is then drawn into a microscopic needle and is injected into the egg. The entire procedure is performed using microscopic instrumentation under robotic control while being visualized through a video camera attached to a microscope.

If fertilization occurs, two pronuclei (small circles in the center of the fertilized egg, containing the combined genetic material from both the egg and the sperm) will become visible within 16-18 hours after the injection. Cell division will occur approximately 12 hours later. At this point of development, the embryo is at the two-cell stage. Frequently, embryos created via ICSI look "healthier" than those created via natural (IVF) fertilization. **Unfortunately, the genetic quality of an embryo cannot be predicted on the basis of the embryo's appearance.**

Experience has shown that normal fertilization and pregnancy rates can be achieved with ICSI even with sperm that are morphologically abnormal (irregularly shaped). These findings challenge the long-held belief that abnormally shaped sperm are likely to be genetically impaired and thus incapable of fertilizing an egg. They also challenge the concept that surgery is the only treatment option for a man with an abnormal sperm count thought to be related to a varicocele—a varicose vein in the testicle that is alleged to cause male infertility through the production of abnormally shaped sperm.

Because ICSI results in such high fertilization rates, we use the technique if we suspect for any reason that a male's sperm will be incapable of fertilizing his partner's eggs. We base these suspicions on such factors as poor fertilization rates during a previous IVF cycle, poor post-processing velocity of the sperm specimen, eggs with a thickened zona pellucida or a high proportion of sperm that appear to be abnormally shaped. Likewise, since fertilization failure may ultimately be the cause of some couples' unexplained infertility, I believe that at least 50% of their eggs should be treated with ICSI to ensure that some of them will fertilize. In my practice, I prefer to err on the side of being aggressive and perform ICSI on the day of the retrieval whenever it appears possible that the process of natural fertilization may be compromised. Using ICSI proactively gives patients the best chance for a successful outcome, since the highest possible number of eggs will be fertilized and a greater number of embryos will be created. With more embryos available for transfer, there is a higher probability for conception. It is not difficult to imagine the emotional devastation that a couple experiences when they are informed that there has been a total lack of fertilization. Fortunately, the use of ICSI has made such scenarios a rare occurrence.

ASSISTED HATCHING

Six or seven days after fertilization, at the blastocyst stage, when the embryo has undergone numerous cell divisions and contains thousands of cells within the zona pellucida, the zona must break to allow the embryo to implant into the uterine lining. This process is exactly like a baby chick breaking out of the shell of its egg. Certain patients, however, produce embryos that appear to be viable but are unable to break out of the zona. These patients may benefit from assisted hatching. In this micromanipulation technique, the embryologist thins areas of the zona pellucida using a microscopic laser or the microscopic application of very dilute acidic enzyme to the embryos' surface. This procedure, which thins the zona pellucida, is performed when the embryo is at the 8-cell stage or later, just before the embryo transfer.

Assisted hatching may be used in patients who have

abnormally thick zonas or have failed to achieve pregnancy despite transfers of healthy-looking embryos in previous cycles. The use of this technique has also been advocated for older women in hopes that it will contribute to increasing pregnancy rates.

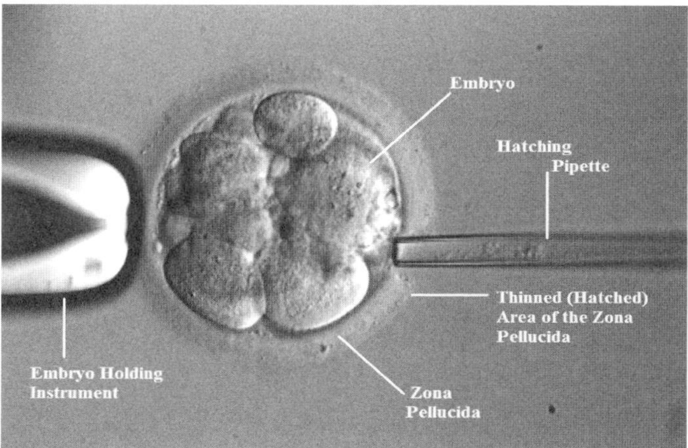

Fig. 5. ***Assisted hatching of an embryo prior to transfer.***

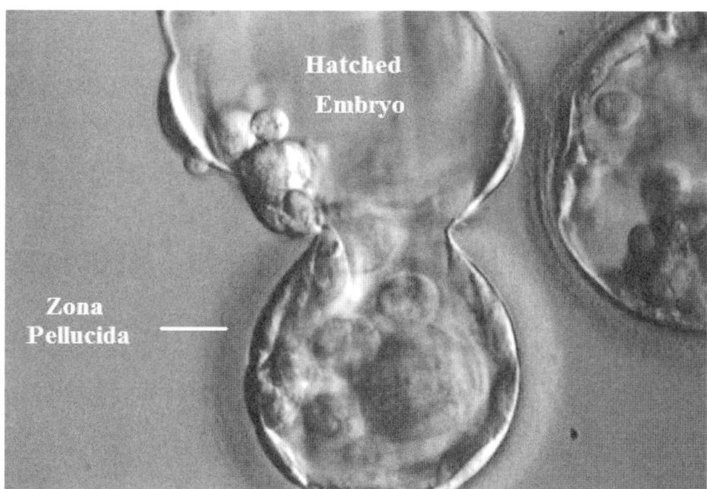

Fig. 6. ***Embryo hatching out of its shell, the zona pellucida.***

THE EMBRYO TRANSFER

TIMING

Once fertilization has taken place, the embryo transfer may occur anywhere from one to six days later. In the early years of IVF, embryo transfer was always performed after two days, at the 2-and-4-cell stage. The laboratory expertise had not yet been developed to allow a developing embryo to survive outside a woman's body for a longer period.

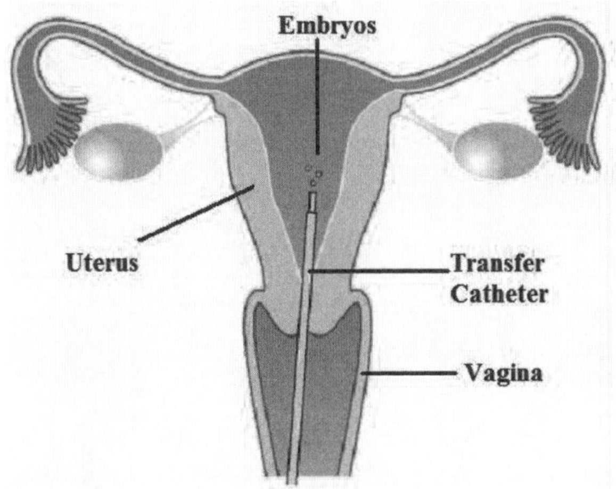

Fig. 7. ***Schematic of an Embryo Transfer.***

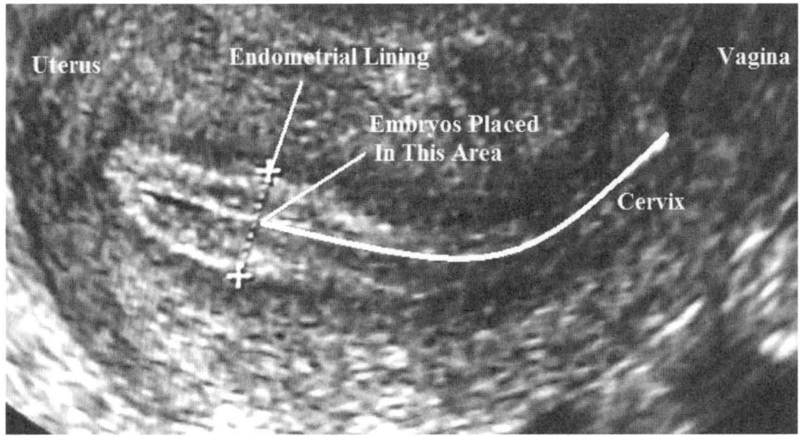

Fig. 8. ***Embryo Transfer: sonographic view of the uterus prior to the actual placement of the embryos***

Thanks to improved culture media and techniques, embryos can now be sustained in a tissue culture environment for a much longer period of time than was previously possible. Today, the majority of IVF centers routinely transfer embryos at 72 hours instead of 24-48 hours. In addition to allowing the uterine lining to develop more fully, this additional time allows the embryologist to evaluate the embryos as they develop. Some eggs may fertilize initially, but then the embryo might stop dividing between the 2- and 6-cell stage. Other embryos may divide too slowly. If an embryo is incapable of reaching at least the 6-cell, if not the 8-cell stage, by day 3, it is a sign that it may be of poor quality and will not develop into a viable pregnancy. In our experience, however, we have occasionally seen a viable pregnancy result from the transfer of a single 4-cell embryo on day 3. The critical fact is that the prediction of a successful pregnancy cannot be based entirely on the appearance of an embryo or its growth rate. In fact, a minimum of 40-50%

of perfect-appearing embryos from a young woman may be genetically abnormal. Irrespective of how the embryos look at time of transfer, all bets are off until the result of the pregnancy test is revealed!

Another advantage to culturing embryos for three days is that the embryos can be observed to see if any of their cells break apart instead of multiplying normally. This is called blastomere fragmentation. If a blastomere is abnormal it may fragment and self-destruct, whereas genetically normal blastomeres continue to grow. The degree of embryo fragmentation, which is factored into the designation of "embryo quality," is considered a reflection of its likelihood for implantation. However, the absence of fragmentation does not guarantee that an embryo will become a viable pregnancy, nor does a significant degree of fragmentation preclude the possibility that an embryo will implant. This is because genetically abnormal blastomeres can remain intact without fragmenting. As long as there is one genetically normal blastomere in an embryo, the possibility of pregnancy exists. No matter what degree of fragmentation is found in an embryo, the fragments can be removed at the time of Assisted Hatching. Removing fragments allows for more room within the embryo for the healthier blastomeres to continue dividing.

BLASTOCYST CULTURE AND TRANSFER

Currently, the state of the art of embryo culture is growing the embryos for five to six days, at which point they should reach the blastocyst stage. This advancement was made possible by defining new culture mediums that allow the embryos to continue to grow in the laboratory for an extra two days. The significance of this development is that prolonged culture will further weed out embryos that appear normal on day 3 at the 8-cell stage, but will fail to develop into normal blastocysts by day 5 or 6.

The length of embryo culture and the timing of the transfer depend on the number of embryos available for transfer and the age of the patient. Blastocyst culture is useful as an embryo sorting strategy to help younger women who produce large numbers of high-fertility potential embryos maximize their chance for a single pregnancy. Since extended culture may help sort out the good embryos from the slower-growing ones, it allows for the selection and transfer of the embryos most likely to result in a pregnancy. In this subgroup of patients it may be helpful in reducing a couple's risk of having a multiple pregnancy. For example, consider the case of a 25-year-old woman who produced 20 eggs during an IVF cycle, 18 of which fertilized. On day 3, there were 13 perfectly formed 8-cell embryos. If no more than two embryos should be transferred for fear of a multiple birth, how is the embryo selection process best managed? One plan is randomly to select two embryos to transfer and freeze the remaining 11, knowing that many of them would not continue to grow and have the possibility of becoming a viable pregnancy. Another approach would be to allow all the embryos to grow in culture for an additional two days to the point at which the ones with the most potential for pregnancy would develop into normal blastocysts, while the others would fall by the wayside. In this case, five of the thirteen 8-cell embryos became fully developed blastocysts. This means that eight embryos, which were thought to have been of good quality, were eliminated by the process of natural selection. Two embryos were selected for transfer, and the remaining three were cryopreserved for future use.

Although an embryo may reach the blastocyst stage, it does not guarantee that it will be genetically perfect. In fact, even in younger women, as many as 50% of blastocysts may contain an abnormal chromosomal complement. Therefore, it is not surprising that a significantly higher percentage of blastocysts derived from women over the age of 35 will be genetically abnormal. I believe that for this group of patients it is preferable to transfer four or five 8-cell embryos on day 3 and let natural selection operate in the uterus rather than incurring the extra expense of blastocyst culture or PGD.

THE PROCEDURE

Transferring embryos into a woman's uterine cavity is the easiest element of IVF, but it is also the most critical. Abdominal ultrasound is used to visualize the transfer, since precise placement cannot be guaranteed unless the doctor can see the exact location of the catheter as it is inserted and watch the embryos as they are deposited into the uterus. Otherwise, the embryos could become transferred too low down in the uterus—or they might not make it into the uterine cavity at all.

The patient starts out with a mildly full bladder, which is necessary for a clear abdominal ultrasound picture. The doctor inserts a speculum into the woman's vagina and cleans her cervix. A plastic tube is then passed through the woman's cervix into the lower part of the uterine cavity. The embryologist picks up the embryos in the smallest amount of fluid (transfer medium) possible and brings them into the procedure room. The catheter is threaded through the outer plastic tubing the doctor has inserted and is advanced 1/2 to 3/4 inch behind the outer sheath. The embryos are then gently injected into the uterine cavity. Since air bubbles in the transfer medium can be seen via ultrasound, it is possible to watch the placement of the embryos on the video monitor.

After placement, the catheter must be removed slowly and gently, since too-rapid removal might create suction that could draw the embryos out of the uterus. Once the catheter has been withdrawn, the embryologist checks it under the microscope to ensure that none of the embryos has stuck to its plastic surface. Should this happen (a rare occurrence) they would be returned to the uterus—but in a lower position, so as not to interfere with those embryos that have already been transferred.

AFTER THE TRANSFER

Every couple undergoing IVF needs to understand that it is virtually impossible for the embryos to "fall out" of the uterine cavity due to insufficient rest or excessive activity following the transfer. The implantation process is out of the couple's control; if an embryo fails to implant, the cause is almost certainly genetic rather than mechanical. There is nothing either the doctor or the couple can do to make a genetically abnormal embryo "stick." This includes the so-called embryo glue, which is hyaluranic acid—a biological enzyme that is added to the transfer medium in the hope that it will aid in embryo hatching and implantation.

It is recommended that patients rest for 30 minutes after the transfer and as much as possible for the remainder of the day. Thereafter, normal activities, including light exercise, are permissible. No evidence exists to suggest that prolonged bed rest or the avoidance of exercise and sexual activity will aid in conception. In fact, some research studies indicate that the pregnancy rates are the same whether patients stay in bed for two weeks after the embryo transfer or immediately resume their normal activities.

POST-TRANSFER MEDICATIONS

After the transfer, the woman will usually be advised to take supplemental progesterone to assist the embryo implant. Progesterone can be administered via intramuscular injection, vaginal suppositories, cream or tablets. We do not use the intramuscular form of progesterone because it is painful to inject and it may cause abscesses at the injection site. Occasionally, the woman will be instructed to take a small dose of HCG every three days to help the ovary produce additional progesterone. Supplemental HCG can stimulate ovarian hyperstimulation syndrome and give a false-positive pregnancy test. Since it takes HCG five days to be cleared from the body, no pregnancy test should be taken before at least five days after the final injection.

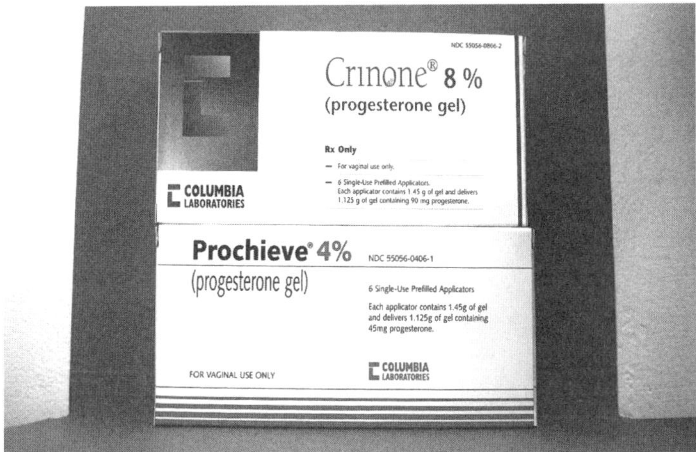

Fig. 9A. ***The various forms of progesterone that is taken to support the luteal phase. I prefer using vaginal progesterone since the hormone is absorbed into the tissues directly, in close proximity to the uterus, where it is needed. Vaginal progesterone can be given in gel, tablet or suppository form. They are all equally effective.***

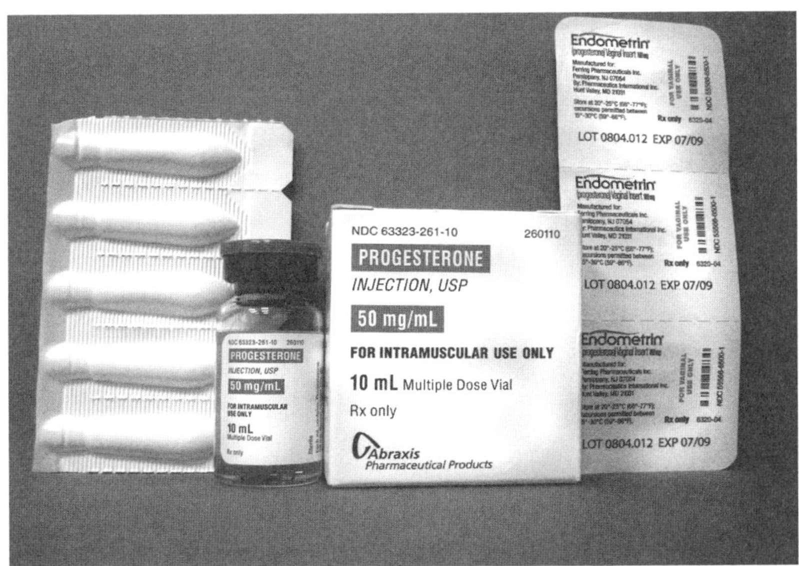

Fig. 9B. ***Progesterone suppositories and injectable Progesterone. Progesterone treatment after embryo transfer is especially important when lupron is part of the stimulation protocol.***

THE WAITING PERIOD

The waiting period between the embryo transfer and the initial pregnancy test seems to take forever. All couples experience varying degrees of emotional turmoil during this time, ranging from high levels of anxiety to insatiable curiosity. The high levels of progesterone that are taken may make matters worse for many women. Nevertheless, I urge patients not to take their first pregnancy test until 10-12 days after the embryo transfer to reduce the probability of false-positive results stemming from residual HGC, which can stay in the system for five to seven days after being injected. False negative results can occur if the blood test is taken before the embryo starts producing detectable levels of HCG, the pregnancy hormone, since some embryos take a few more days to implant than others. Although urine pregnancy tests are accurate, they are significantly less sensitive than are the blood tests.

Since there is no evidence that bed rest affects the probability of conception, the time will pass much more quickly if the woman remains active and productive during this period. Both partners should do whatever they can to reduce their stress levels and focus on other aspects in their lives during this difficult period.

Although every couple needs to decide for themselves whether to tell friends and family about their infertility treatment, many women who have undergone the process report that a significant source of stress during the two-week post-transfer period comes from well-meaning friends and family members who ask "how things are going?" Even if the couple has been successful in refocusing their own attentions during this period, the interest of others may rekindle their obsession as to whether or not the woman has conceived.

One option for couples that choose to discuss their treatment with others is to do so only in general terms, without divulging the exact dates of procedures. This may save them the stress of having to respond repeatedly, to such questions as "Do you feel pregnant?" or "Did you get your period yet?"

IF THE IVF CYCLE IS NOT SUCCESSFUL

In deciding what course of action to recommend to couples who have had an unsuccessful IVF cycle, the doctor needs to take into account the woman's age, her response to the medication, the quality and fertilization rate of her eggs, whether any embryos reached the blastocyst stage and whether the couple has had any embryos frozen for future use. Based on this information, the doctor may suggest that the couple try IVF treatment again, with a change in the drug protocol, or try a completely different course of action. The couple then needs to consider the doctor's recommendation in terms of their own financial and emotional reserves, along with their level of commitment to the goal of creating a biological child.

CRYOPRESERVATION (FREEZING) OF EXTRA EMBRYOS

The technology that enables us to preserve living cells for an indefinite period of time may sound like science fiction, but it actually was developed many years ago, in the 1960s. We are not referring to the freezing of an entire human body, which is obviously impossible, but to certain types of live single cell units, namely sperm and embryos. The cryopreservation of unfertilized eggs is a much newer and more complex development. In the early 1980s the first baby was born from a frozen embryo and, since that time, a 100,000 or more babies derived from frozen embryos have been born worldwide.

The technology was originally developed in the animal breeding industry, so that sperm from prize animals could be frozen and transported for insemination into receptive females worldwide. A single frozen bull sperm specimen could be used to fertilize many cows. This was more efficient and lucrative than having the animals mate the "old-fashioned" way!

The technique of freezing embryos, which is quite different from that of freezing sperm, was also developed in the cattle breeding industry. In this case, a prized cow was given fertility drugs to produce multiple eggs and was then fertilized naturally. In cows, but unfortunately not in humans, embryos can be nonsurgically removed from the uterus prior to their implantation. The multiple embryos obtained from a single cow are then frozen and, at a later date, transferred into several ordinary cows that will carry the pregnancy to term. Because of the ability to cryopreserve embryos, many more cattle can be born as the result of a single breeding session.

Just as the cryopreservation of embryos makes animal breeding much more efficient, it is also advantageous for human reproduction. In many cases, women who are high responders will produce many eggs and, subsequently, many more embryos than could safely be transferred in one IVF cycle. The ability to preserve extra embryos in a frozen state is obviously useful to a couple trying to conceive with IVF. When conception occurs after the transfer of fresh embryos, the remaining cryopreserved embryos can be used several years later in an attempt to conceive another child without having to undergo the entire IVF procedure. A frozen embryo transfer cycle is much easier for a patient compared with an IVF cycle in terms of medication, monitoring, procedures and expense. Moreover, embryos harvested from a woman when she was 32 years old have a greater chance of creating a pregnancy than do embryos created from eggs harvested when she is several years older. It is important to note that there is no time limit or "expiration date" for embryos to remain in the frozen state. In fact, one of my patients returned for the transfer of frozen embryos ten years after the birth of twins from an IVF cycle. Two out of three frozen embryos survived after being thawed. The woman conceived and delivered a baby, which was technically a fraternal triplet to its eleven-year-old siblings!

The same advantage exists for a patient when conception does not occur with the transfer of fresh embryos. The fact that several embryos remain in a frozen state for another attempt at conception gives a couple some encouragement despite their disappointment that the current cycle did not work. On the other hand, when women are in their late thirties or when their ovarian reserve is low, couples should not anticipate having extra embryos left over for cryopreservation.

Most people would assume that embryos and sperm are frozen by the same methods that are used to freeze food, and are stored in a freezer. Nothing can be further from the truth! As living entities, sperm must retain the ability to swim and embryos must be able to continue to grow after being thawed from the frozen state. The trick is to keep the interior of the cells, which contain water, from forming ice crystals during the freezing process. When ice crystals form inside the cell, the interior implodes and results in cell death. In the case of sperm, prior to freezing in liquid nitrogen (-273 degrees F), ice crystallization is prevented by the addition of glycerol, which is actually a component of antifreeze. The sperm are frozen in thin straws or small vials and stored in tanks containing liquid nitrogen.

The cryopreservation of embryos is a more complex process. In order to prevent intracellular ice crystallization, the embryos are immersed in a series of sugar solutions that draw out all the water from inside the cell. If there is no water, then there can be no ice formed inside. The embryos are placed in thin straws, in which they are frozen and stored in liquid nitrogen. Embryos can be frozen at all stages—from the single cell pronucleate stage to the blastocyst stage. Each embryonic stage requires a different freezing protocol. A new freezing technique, a process called vitrification, shows great promise in the cryopreservation of both embryos and unfertilized oocytes.

CRYOPRESERVATION OF UNFERTILIZED EGGS

The freezing of unfertilized eggs is a more difficult task. Eggs that have not yet been fertilized are much more fragile than fertilized eggs and do not survive the process nearly as well. Embryos survive the freezing process 80-85% of the time; unfertilized oocytes survive with significantly less frequency. The relatively few that do survive the freeze/thaw cycle must then be fertilized successfully and develop into embryos. To further complicate matters, eggs that have been cryopreserved do not fertilize naturally, but require that a sperm be injected inside with ICSI. Fertilization rates are far lower after cryopreservation than with eggs that are fertilized after retrieval. This is due to the fact that freezing, more often than not, disturbs the spindle mechanism that actually joins the chromosomes from the egg and the sperm together. If the chromosomes do not unite, fertilization is impossible.

There are several areas in which it would be quite useful to cryopreserve unfertilized eggs. In unfortunate instances when a young woman requires chemotherapy or pelvic radiation to treat a malignancy, these treatments almost always will be toxic to her eggs and will render her sterile. Should such a patient not have a male partner at the time, the ability to save her unfertilized egg for future use would enable her to have her own biological child at a later date.

Because today's couples are marrying later in life—in many cases in their late 30s or early 40s, infertility due to advanced maternal age is a distinct possibility. It would be a great advantage for women to be able to save their eggs in their early 20s, when the oocytes are still of high quality, as an "insurance policy" against age-related infertility. The technology is readily available, but the cost of the procedure, which is not covered by insurance, and the fact that most women in their 20s assume that they are "eternally fertile," cause elective oocyte cryopreservation to be requested infrequently. Most of the patients who ask me about saving their eggs are between 35 and 42 years old and are not actually appropriate candidates for this procedure. Because both egg reserve and quality decline with increasing age, the chance of pregnancy resulting from cryopreserved eggs is small. In fact, the American Society of Reproductive Medicine specifically recommends against oocyte cryopreservation after the age of 35.

Young people in the modern world seem to me to be in a difficult situation. Couples marrying in their early 20s do not generally have a high rate of infertility, but do have an increasingly high divorce rate. Couples that marry later in life may make better choices in selecting a mate, but statistically have a very high rate of infertility. With the age of adulthood in Generations X and Y being defined as 30 years old, marriage will undoubtedly be later for the vast majority of young Americans. Infertility will become an even greater problem, which will have far-reaching consequences in population growth and economic conditions. As far as I can see, there is no solution to this conundrum.

CLINICAL CASE STUDIES: *IN VITRO* FERTILIZATION

CASE #1: CAROLINE AND JOE

Caroline, a 34-year-old anesthesiologist, had been trying to conceive for three years. She had never given birth but had an early, uncomplicated abortion at age 20. Her diagnostic workup was completely normal but her husband, Joe (47), was found to have a very low sperm count, with abnormally shaped sperm and poor post-processing velocity. He was never able to father a child, despite having tried for many years during a previous marriage. The working diagnosis for the couple was severe male-factor infertility. Since Joe's sperm was in the 2-4 million range, the couple was advised to skip IUI and proceed directly to IVF with ICSI. They agreed.

During their first IVF cycle, Caroline responded well to stimulation with Lupron and FSH and produced 14, mature-looking eggs. But when the embryologist stripped the eggs to prepare them for ICSI, they were all found to be in Metaphase I and too immature to be fertilized, even though HCG had been given 36 hours earlier. The eggs were allowed additional time to mature in the lab, but only four went on to reach maturity at the Metaphase II stage; the remainder never matured. The embryologist performed ICSI on the four mature eggs, but only one embryo developed. This embryo was able to reach only the 6-cell stage before the transfer and there was also some fragmentation. Sadly, Caroline did not become pregnant.

Although Joe had always believed that he bore the sole responsibility for the couple's failure to conceive, it now appeared that an underlying problem with Caroline's eggs was a significant part of their failure to conceive. The doctor advised the couple to repeat IVF in several months with a different stimulation protocol, to see if the quality of Caroline's eggs could be improved. If the same problem were to occur on the second try, and if the couple remained committed to trying for a pregnancy, he would suggest that they consider IVF with donor eggs.

CASE #2: IVF AND UNEXPLAINED INFERTILITY—BARBARA AND JONAS

This young couple married in their early 20s and did not conceive after five years of having unprotected sex. Both the male and female infertility evaluations were normal. The couple had tried the usual six cycles of controlled ovarian hyperstimulation, combined with intrauterine insemination, without success.

The couple was optimistic that a pregnancy would result from IVF on the first attempt. I cautioned them not to be too hopeful with the first IVF treatment because couples with a long-standing history of unexplained infertility may sometimes have an egg-quality issue, which has a guarded prognosis. Rather, I suggested that they focus on the diagnostic value of the first IVF cycle because it would enable us to observe directly the condition of Barbara's eggs, the rate of their fertilization and the quality of the embryos that are produced.

As expected, the stimulation was excellent and Barbara produced 23 eggs, 19 of which appeared to be mature. Nine of the eggs were allowed to fertilize naturally, of which three actually fertilized. Of the ten oocytes that were to be fertilized with ICSI, on closer inspection, seven were mature. Only three eggs fertilized. Barbara's fertilization rate was only 26% (6/23), which was significantly lower than normal. Of the six fertilized eggs, two reached the 8-cell stage by the third day of growth in the lab. Both had between 10% and 20% fragmentation. The other embryos' growth was arrested at the 2-4-cell stage and therefore had died before transfer. When an analysis of the couple's cycle was performed, it was not surprising to learn that there was no conception.

This case illustrates the important diagnostic value of an IVF cycle. Although they were disappointed that pregnancy did not occur, they learned that Jonas' sperm could fertilize Barbara's eggs naturally. This was a great relief to them, as it was one of their major concerns. Their problem seemed to be one of an egg factor. None of the many eggs that Barbara produced was good enough to produce a pregnancy. This couple may choose to try another IVF cycle with a different drug protocol in the future, hoping that she will produce better-quality eggs and embryos with different medications. Barbara and Jonas could also decide to continue trying to conceive naturally, since they learned that her eggs could be fertilized without assistance, patiently waiting for the month that the perfect egg and sperm unite to form a viable conception. Their chances of conception naturally may be just as good as with any form of fertility treatment. Since Barbara is only 26 years old and has an excellent egg reserve, the couple need not worry about age as a factor contributing pressure to conceive quickly. The couple's other options are using donor oocytes or adoption, depending entirely on the immediacy of their need to have a baby.

This case illustrates an important point for all to understand and remember. Although there are no guarantees in life, conception is always possible as long as a woman is under 44 years of age. This explains the fact that 3% of couples that adopt a baby because they are considered "hopelessly infertile," will eventually conceive on their own. This is not because of psychological factors, such as "they were relaxed because the pressure to have a child was removed." Rather, it is the egg factor that causes this phenomenon. If a woman produces 12 eggs per year, and it takes her five years to become pregnant, then 1/60 or 1.06% of her eggs are genetically perfect enough to create a viable pregnancy. Although a 1.06% chance of conception may seem very low, it is not 0% and it is far better than the chance of winning the lottery!

SUMMARY

IVF is the ultimate diagnostic tool available today. It provides a firsthand look at your eggs and embryos, in order to find any subtle or unanticipated problems that may exist on a cellular level. The procedure provides the best opportunity to diagnose what might be otherwise undetectable causes of infertility. At the same time, IVF is the only diagnostic procedure that offers a couple an optimal chance to conceive.

With the development of ICSI, the treatment of male infertility has been revolutionized. Even men who produce only the smallest numbers of sperm now have the chance to achieve fatherhood.

Since IVF (with or without ICSI) works best in couples in which the woman is as close to her "biological prime" as possible, don't let anyone try to convince you that you are too young for these techniques. Withholding these most potent and direct cures for infertility in the mistaken belief that a relatively young couple should work toward a "natural" conception is both illogical and counterproductive. IVF is a safe, non-invasive procedure that can help you conceive by bypassing tubal disorders, ovulation problems and many undetectable causes of unexplained infertility.

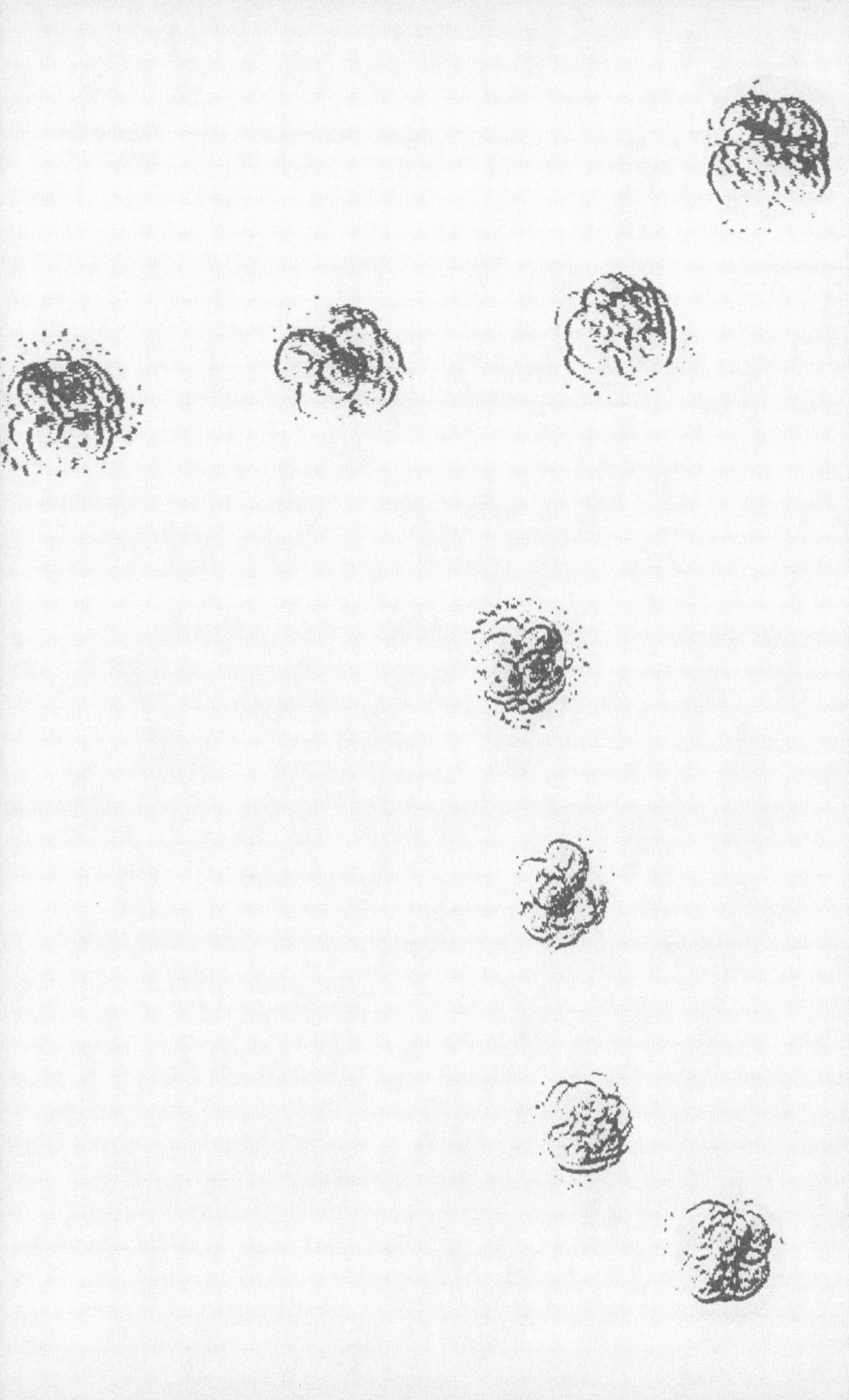

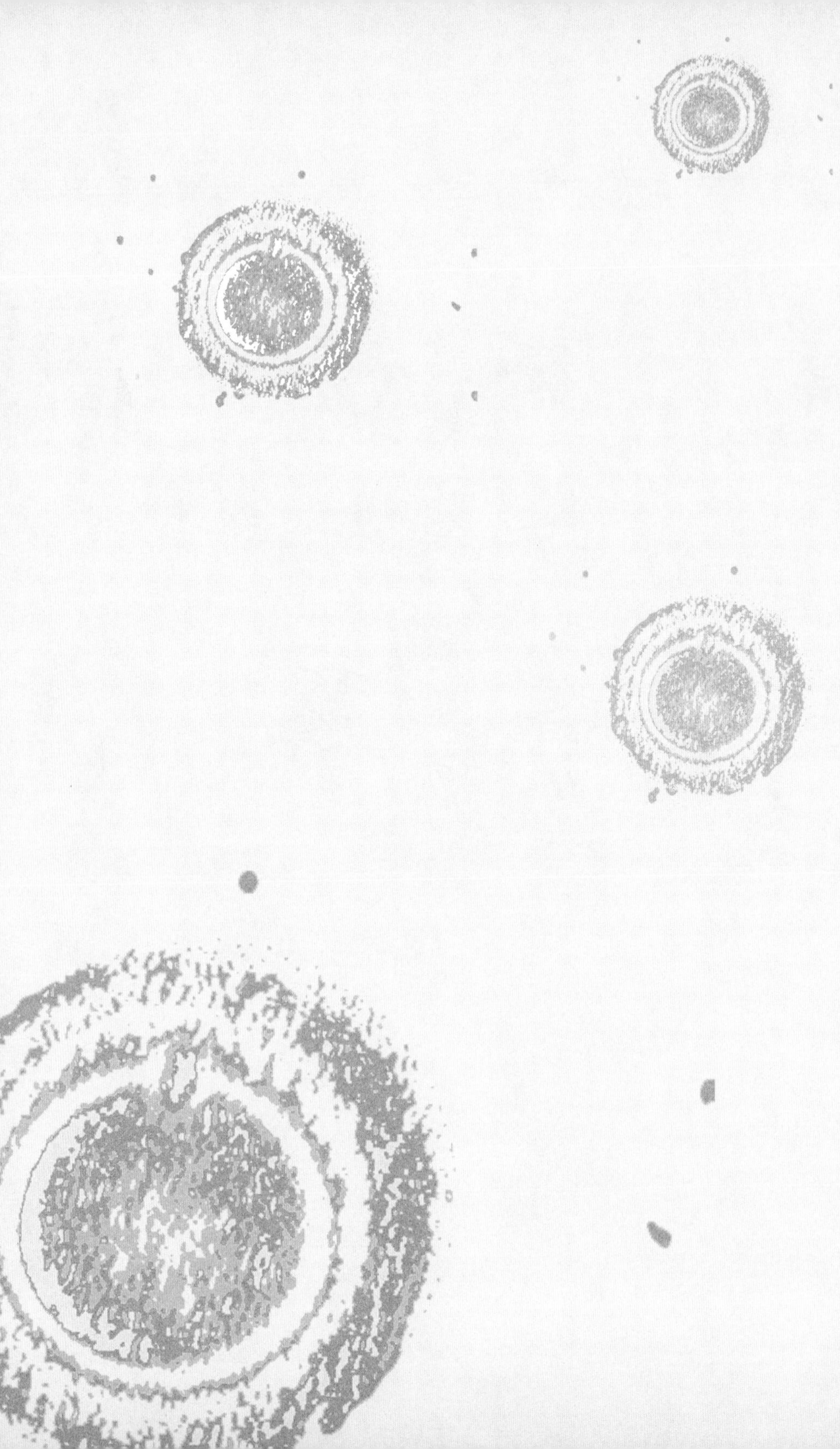

CHAPTER 11

STEP 4
IVF with Donor Eggs and Gestational Surrogacy

Having read the first two chapters in this book, you can readily appreciate why a woman's age is the most important factor in predicting the likelihood of conception. Beyond a certain age (which differs for every woman), the vast majority of eggs will have genetically deteriorated to such an extent that conception may become impossible. This point in time may actually occur five to ten years before the onset of menopause, while the woman still gets regular periods, has normal FSH levels and may even have a moderate amount of eggs left in her ovaries. When this scenario occurs, IVF with donor eggs may offer the only chance for a pregnancy. The use of eggs donated from a young woman to an older one is the only available way to turn back the "biological clock."

The use of donated eggs is actually a tissue transplant. For example, when an individual's kidneys cease to function, the possibility of receiving a healthy kidney from a donor is a life-saving option. Similarly, when a woman's oocytes are of poor quality or are depleted, using oocytes derived from a donor is a viable option to have a child. Just as a kidney from a donor, which is genetically different from the recipient's own tissues, becomes the functioning kidney of the recipient after it has been transplanted, any baby born as a result of using donated eggs is the offspring of the birth mother. **The law is very clear in stating that the woman giving birth to a baby is its legal mother and, as such, her name appears on the baby's birth certificate**. Furthermore, the law specifically states that any individual who donates eggs or sperm has no parental rights to reclaim a child conceived with their donated reproductive tissues. Therefore, there should be no concern that a donor may appear at a later date and attempt to take a baby away from its legal mother.

Fortunately, the process of egg donation is much easier for the recipient, compared with an individual receiving an organ transplant. No blood or tissue typing is necessary to match an egg donor with a recipient nor are any toxic immunosuppressive drugs required. This is possible because the uterus is an immunologically "privileged" site. The uterus is unique in that genetically foreign tissue can grow in it without the body's immune defense mechanisms attacking and destroying it. Since every fetus is genetically different from its mother due to the father's genetic contribution, an exception to the universal laws of immune rejection of genetically foreign tissues is essential for the propagation of the human race!

It may take a bit of time to become comfortable with the concept of attempting conception with eggs donated by an genetically unrelated woman. In order to address some of the concerns couples normally have regarding egg donation, the way in which physical characteristics and other traits are inherited must be understood. The most important concept to appreciate is that, unlike a person's body cells, which all contain identical DNA molecules, the DNA in each and every egg and sperm cell is slightly different. In actuality, each egg and sperm contains unique DNA material contributed by each one of our ancestors, going back to prehistoric times. This is the precise reason why each member of a family has a unique physical appearance, while at the same time, shares similar features and characteristics with other individuals in their family. For instance, a man may have his father's muscular body type, his mother's wavy blond hair and his paternal great aunt's unusually light green eyes. He is, however, considerably shorter than all other family members. When he examined his family tree, he was surprised to find out that his maternal great-grandfather was unusually short.

A further example is the case of fraternal twins. They are the product of two different sperm and eggs and are always quite different in appearance, yet bear some degree of resemblance to each other. These differences are the result of the different DNA content of each egg and sperm cell. Simply stated, when a couple has a large family, all the children are quite different in appearance and none is ever an exact "clone" of either parent. Therefore, as long as a donor is chosen who has similar physical characteristics to that of the recipient, the baby conceived with that donor's eggs and the husband's sperm will, in a general way, have an appearance that is in harmony with the rest of the family.

Unfortunately, some couples are fixated on obtaining eggs from a donor with certain specific characteristics and abilities. For instance, several years ago I met with a high-power couple that was willing to pay $50,000 to obtain eggs from a six-foot-tall, blond, Harvard student having an IQ of no less than 150. They failed to understand that each of the donor's eggs could produce a baby with quite different characteristics. It is very possible that the donor had an ancestor who was very short in stature and was of only average intelligence whose genetic material was contained in one of her eggs. If that egg, of all the others that she produced, was the one that resulted in that couple's baby, they would have a child that would be far different from their fantasy. If, in fact, the baby born to such a couple were not tall, blond, beautiful and brilliant, how would they treat that child? I, personally, would have great concerns that such a couple could possibly reject any child that did not meet their expectations. As such, my inclination is to strongly discourage couples looking for a "designer" baby from considering parenthood.

WHO ARE THE EGG DONORS?

Women choose to become anonymous egg donors for a variety of reasons. Some have no current interest in becoming pregnant and believe that their eggs are "going to waste." Others donate for truly altruistic purposes, wanting to help couples that are desperate to conceive. Many donors have friends or relatives who are infertile and donate because they are empathic to the plight of couples who are unable to conceive. Most commonly, the donors rely on the standard $8,000 stipend to help support their families or pay for their education. Such motivation is both legitimate and reasonable for the effort, risks, discomfort and inconvenience that they endure. Donors who demand excessive compensation should not be used; they often prove to be unreliable and are generally difficult to work with. Needless to say, women who donate their eggs offer a priceless gift to couples that have nowhere else to turn in their quest to have a baby.

Anonymous egg donors are usually recruited by an infertility clinic via word-of-mouth or through advertisements placed in college papers, as a service for their patients. Patients are usually not charged an extra fee for this service. There are also agencies that recruit donors, but their administrative recruitment fees will usually add $10,000-15,000 to the cost of the egg donation cycle. Occasionally, a known donor, either a relative or a close friend, will volunteer to donate her eggs without compensation. It is important to remember that all egg donors, either anonymous or known, should be under 30 years of age in order to provide eggs of the highest genetic quality.

Potential egg donors typically undergo an extensive series of interviews to determine their suitability to participate in an oocyte donation program. Appropriate motivation and the ability to be fully cognizant of all the aspects of the medical process, including all potential side effects and complications, are key elements in determining whether a candidate can be considered for donor screening. Also essential is the capability and willingness to self-administer daily injections and to have frequent blood tests and sonograms. Women who are interested only in financial compensation are not selected, since experience has shown them to be unreliable. We receive frequent calls from young women, saying that they will be visiting New York City for a few days and would like to "sell some of their eggs". Obviously, such individuals cannot be considered as potential egg donors, since their motivation is inappropriate and they having no understanding of the medical process. If a donor applicant has multiple body piercings and tattoos they may be rejected since egg donation is prohibited if their "body art" is recent because they are at some risk to have been exposed to the hepatitis virus. Women who are from countries (England, France) that have had outbreaks of the "Mad Cow Disease" in the human population are excluded from being egg donors in the U.S. by Public Health law.

AN EGG DONATION STORY

Very recently, my wife called my attention to an article about one woman's experience with egg donation, which appeared in a fashion magazine. This article illustrated how intelligent people do not understand basic facts about egg donor selection. The author, a very educated and affluent woman, sought to find an egg donor who would be an ideal match for her. She was not looking to create a "designer baby" but was very earnest in selecting a donor that carried genetic traits that would be compatible with her son, her husband and herself. Not only was she looking for a similarity in physical features, but also in specific intellectual and personality traits. She approached her quest for an egg donor most diligently, viewing donor profiles from many different agencies. She likened her experience to selecting a "dream date" at a dating agency. She even employed an infertility psychologist to help her evaluate potential candidates. ***I found it amazing that she went through this exhaustive and costly quest in order to find a suitable donor without any of the physicians, psychologists and donor agency counselors telling her that each of the donor's eggs contains different genetic material that might produce a child that was quite different from the donor.*** In fact, the agencies seemed to be marketing their donors on the basis of their physical and intellectual characteristics. Such marketing encourages potential recipients to create fantasies about their future babies, which are potentially unrealistic and might lead them to an egg donor who would not be ideal in terms of egg production or quality. In fact some donors demand much higher fees for their eggs because they may be very beautiful, talented or intelligent. Such attempts at commercialization and profiteering by agencies and egg donors should be strongly condemned.

Unfortunately, the donor that the author selected turned out to be a disappointment. The author had arranged to meet her donor after the egg retrieval (which seems to be legal in California) and was disappointed, as the donor's personality and appearance were not exactly what she had imagined. The biggest disappointment, however, was that the donor's eggs, and the subsequent quality of the embryos, were poor. Conception did not occur during the fresh cycle and, despite obtaining 16 eggs, no embryos were available for cryopreservation. I believe that the author's unfortunate experience was a result of a common misconception that an individual can exert control over the genetic processes involved in conception. Individuals can no more control the appearance and characteristics of their dream baby than can a fertility specialist guarantee a conception after implanting a perfectly appearing embryo in a woman's uterus. Conception is too complex a process to be controlled by human efforts and desires. Couples considering egg donation should not focus on superficialities when choosing a donor. Rather, youth, good health, freedom from genetic diseases and excellent ovarian reserve are the key factors in choosing an egg donor.

DONOR SELECTION AND SCREENING

Once a young woman is deemed to be a good candidate for egg donation, the next step is the completion of her biographical, medical and family history questionnaires. Important issues in the personal medical history relate to factors that might pose health risks for the donor or any genetically transmitted medical conditions that could be transferred via her eggs to the recipient's baby. For example, if a candidate has a medical history of juvenile diabetes, she should not be an egg donor since there is potential (though very low) risk to her health and the distinct possibility that her diabetic condition could be passed on to any offspring conceived with her eggs. Other factors that would disqualify a potential donor are extremes in body weight and a history of absent or irregular menstrual periods or the polycystic ovarian syndrome. Very thin women, especially those who menstruate infrequently, are at high risk for the Ovarian Hyperstimulation Syndrome. This may place the donor at high risk for serious medical complications. The same is true for women who have the polycystic ovarian syndrome.

Once a donor is deemed to be an acceptable candidate, her fertility potential is evaluated by measuring her FSH, LH and Estradiol levels early in her menstrual cycle, as well as evaluating her ovarian reserve. If she has a high ovarian reserve of eggs and her hormonal levels are low, she will respond well to ovarian stimulation and produce a substantial number of oocytes. Should a candidate's ovarian reserve be on the low side, and her hormonal levels are somewhat elevated, she will not be an ideal egg donor and should not be selected. Not all very young women will be good donors. Recently, a 21-year-old donor candidate was unfortunately found to be in early menopause. Although one can accurately predict whether a donor will produce an adequate quantity of eggs, the egg quality cannot be foretold.

THE LABORATORY TESTING OF EGG DONORS

The laboratory tests that donors must undergo and the frequency of their testing is strictly controlled by the New York Department of Health and The Center for Disease Control. These government agencies issue licenses to all institutions that perform procedures that involve the transplantation of tissue from one individual to another. In order to maintain a tissue transplantation license, an institution undergoes periodic rigorous inspections to insure that donors have all the necessary blood tests so that patients who receive donated tissues do not run the risk of becoming infected with a disease that was transmitted from the donor via contaminated tissue.

Although you may not have realized it, a blood transfusion is the oldest and most frequently performed type of tissue donation. Unfortunately, prior to the development of the currently available blood tests for infectious agents, many sad lessons were learned about the transmission of serious infections such as Hepatitis A, B, and C, as well as the HIV virus. These days, the blood donor, as well as the unit of blood itself, is tested for all possible forms of known blood-borne diseases. This is especially crucial since the transfusion of blood is the most "efficient" way a individual can become infected, since the circulating blood comes in contact with all parts and organs in the body. Infectious agents may be transmitted both in the liquid component of blood (the serum) and also by the white blood cells. When a blood specimen is contaminated and is injected into another's circulatory system, as in a blood transfusion, the chance of infection is high, but never 100%. Similarly, the transplantation of any tissue that is directly connected to the circulatory system, such as the heart, lungs, kidney, and liver, has a relatively higher risk of transmitting an infectious agent than does an egg, which is not connected to any blood vessels. The donation of sperm has been known to transmit hepatitis B and HIV because these viruses are found in the seminal fluid. Although eggs can be exposed to blood cells during retrieval, viral transmission is only a theoretic possibility. To my knowledge, there have been no reports of viral infection transmitted to recipients of donated eggs.

Sexually transmitted diseases

- Various types of the HIV virus
- Hepatitis A, B, and C
- Syphillis
- Gonorrhea and Chlamydia

Genetically transmitted diseases, where appropriate

- Sickle cell anemia (for African Americans)
- Cystic Fibrosis (for all Caucasians)
- Tay Sachs and other related rare genetic diseases found in people of northern European Jewish ancestry

It is important to know if any of the donor's family members suffer (or have suffered) from such conditions as depression or alcohol abuse, or if there is a history of suicide, since these personality traits are thought to be inheritable. Family histories of diabetes, heart problems, and cancer are relatively common in our society, and since the role of heredity in their development is uncertain, recipients should probably not reject a potential donor based only on the incidence of one of these diseases in the family tree. In fact, these diseases are so widespread that almost everyone has the potential to develop at least one in their lifetime, regardless of family history—particularly if they don't take care of themselves. Besides, medical science has developed excellent screening and treatment techniques for many of these illnesses, so even if the baby does go on to develop one of them in middle age, he or she can still go on to live a long, active life.

THE RECIPIENT

Prior to contemplating carrying a pregnancy conceived with donor eggs, any woman who is over 40 years old must have some basic medical tests performed to insure that she is in a good state of health. At minimum, she should have a physical examination with a complete battery of blood tests and an electrocardiogram. A recent mammogram is also important to rule out the presence of a tiny breast lesion, which could be stimulated to grow as a result of the high hormone levels associated with pregnancy. If there are any preexisting medical conditions, there should be a current reevaluation of its status; any implications and potential complications that could be associated with pregnancy should be discussed with the appropriate specialists. If the donor egg recipient is in her late 40's or 50's, as many of today's women are, a cardiac stress test is advised, to rule out the possibility of latent cardiac disease. Women who are obese, or who have preexisting heart disease, diabetes or high blood pressure are at especially high risk for serious medical complications during pregnancy, that could have dire effects on both their unborn child and themselves. Although there is no official age limit for oocyte recipients, careful consideration of a woman's physical condition is probably more important than her chronological age.

THE PROCESS OF OOCYTE DONATION

An oocyte donation cycle should not take more than eight weeks to complete, from the point of the selection of a donor to the time of the recipient's pregnancy test. The first step in the egg donation process is to synchronize the menstrual cycles of donor and recipient. Synchronization is necessary so that the recipient will be ready to receive the embryos that have been created from eggs produced from the donor's IVF cycle and the recipient's partner's sperm.

Women who no longer get their menstrual periods are concerned that they will be unable to be an oocyte recipient. In fact, postmenopausal women are actually easier to synchronize with a donor than are those who menstruate regularly and have equally high pregnancy rates. These patients are typically placed on some form of natural estrogen (pills or skin patches), which stimulates the growth of the uterine lining. Just as in a normal cycle, the lining of the uterus progressively develops over a period of 12-20 days to reach a thickness of 8 to 12 mm. The development of the endometrium is monitored with a biweekly sonogram. From that point in time the recipient is ready to begin progesterone therapy on the day that the donor's oocytes are harvested. The recipient then takes progesterone injections for three to four days in preparation for the embryo transfer and then continues vaginal progesterone until the time of the pregnancy test.

When women who still get their periods require egg donation, their ovulation must be blocked until the donor starts the stimulation phase of the IVF cycle. This is accomplished by treating both donor and recipient with Lupron for a duration of 1-3 weeks until the ovulation of both women is suppressed. Their cycles of are then synchronized such that the recipient's uterus is ready to receive embryos whenever the donor's eggs become mature and are ready for retrieval. The hormone support therapy is identical for all recipients.

FINANCIAL ASPECTS OF EGG DONATION

When patients hear the cost of an egg donation cycle, they are usually quite shocked about how costly it is. Consequently, it is important that prospective recipients understand the individual components of the procedure and the cost of each. The following components of the donor cycle are listed along with the average fee for each.

- Donor compensation $8000
- Donor screening $2000
- Donor medications $3000
- Donor supplemental health insurance $1000
- Donor/recipient synchronization fees $2000
- Retrieval anesthesia $1000
- IVF/donor & recipient fees $8000
- ICSI if male factor $1000
- Embryo cryopreservation $1000

These costs are for a cycle in which a single recipient receives all the donor's eggs. A donor's eggs can also be shared between two recipients. Clinics differ in their policies on the sharing of donor oocytes. There can be some savings since certain of the costs, like the donor's compensation, medications, and screening expenses, can be shared by the two recipient couples. However, since there are two separate IVF cycles happening simultaneously, the shared cycle may cost approximately 30% less than an unshared cycle. The monetary savings with shared oocytes must be weighed against the reduced number of oocytes that will be available for fertilization and cryopreservation, which may, in some cases, have a negative impact on achieving conception.

IF A DONOR CYCLE IS SUCCESSFUL

A woman who conceives via donor eggs should be monitored via blood hormone level testing and ultrasound two weeks after a positive pregnancy test. At that time, it should be possible to determine the number of viable fetuses.

Normally, once a woman has conceived via donor eggs she is no more at risk for complications than any other pregnant woman. ***Amniocentesis, an invasive genetic test routinely advised for pregnant women over the age of 35, is not called for, since the age of the donor (usually under 30), rather than the age of the recipient, is the relevant factor in assessing the chances for genetic abnormality of the fetus.*** Since the risk of losing a pregnancy after amniocentesis is greater than the probability of finding a genetic abnormality in a fetus produced from a young woman's eggs, I advise that this procedure be avoided unless there is some specific sonographic evidence suggesting a genetic problem. Of course, when a woman carrying a donor pregnancy sees her obstetrician, this fact should be made known on confidential basis so that the issue of amniocentesis does not become problematic in the doctor/patient relationship. However, I do advise blood testing at 15 weeks as a non-invasive means of screening for Down's syndrome and neural defects such as spina bifida.

The only other possibility of increased risks for a woman pregnant via donor eggs are related to her age. Any older woman over the age of 40 years will have a higher-than-normal chance of developing complications as high blood pressure (pre-eclampsia) or gestational diabetes during pregnancy, whether their pregnancy resulted from their own eggs or those of a donor. These medical situations are routinely screened for in all pregnant women and are usually recognized at any early stage and can be treated successfully, with a good outcome for both mother and baby. However, these conditions are associated with a higher incidence of prematurity, stillbirth and maternal complications. When an older woman carries twins, her risk of problems is even greater. In the rare case of a woman over 40 conceiving triplets, fetal reduction is recommended since the risks for a fetal or maternal complication are unacceptably high. If a woman over 40 is pregnant, she does not necessarily need to be under the care of a "high risk" obstetrician. If a preexisting medical condition exists, or if a complication develops during a pregnancy, an obstetrician will bring in appropriate medical specialists for consultation and treatment when necessary.

"SHOULD WE TELL?"

One of the most common questions asked by potential recipient couples is whether they should tell friends, family, and ultimately, the child, that their conception was achieved via donor eggs.

Ultimately, each couple must decide for themselves whether or not to share the details of their child's conception. The issue of disclosure is quite different in the case of adoption. It has been clearly shown by a voluminous amount of research that disclosure is advisable so that an adopted child gradually understands and accepts their unique situation. As far as I can tell, there is no firm consensus of opinion about disclosure with regard to egg donation. The vast majority of our recipient couples are strongly against disclosure in order that their offspring be spared the psychological issues that adopted children may struggle with as they grow up. I tend to agree with them, since the less information of this nature the child has, the fewer emotional issues they will have to deal with in the future. However, we advise couples who are leaning toward disclosure to at least wait until after the baby is born to share the information with others. Once a woman has carried a baby for nine months and then gone through childbirth, the origin of the egg becomes truly irrelevant.

If a couple does decide against disclosure, they should follow an "all-or-nothing" rule. If even one other person knows about the egg donation, there will always be the possibility that their confidentiality will be violated. Regardless of their ultimate decision, the couple's obstetrician should be told about the donation since the fact that the egg comes from a younger woman is relevant to the decision as to whether or not an amniocentesis should be performed.

IF A DONOR CYCLE IS NOT SUCCESSFUL

Just as with one's own eggs, achieving a pregnancy with donor eggs is usually a matter of persistence. However, if a particular donor's eggs don't produce a pregnancy after two or three attempts (despite good stimulation and the production of a large number of eggs), the couple should switch to a different donor. The clinic should probably terminate this donor's participation in the program, since the genetic quality of her eggs may have already started to deteriorate. For their second donor, the couple might be well-advised to select a woman whose eggs have created a recent pregnancy.

CLINICAL CASE STUDY: IVF WITH DONOR EGGS

Caroline and Joe, the couple who had unsuccessfully attempted IVF in Chapter 10, remained unable to conceive despite two additional IVF cycles. The doctor urged them to consider donor eggs. Joe was extremely eager to become a father, so he readily agreed. Caroline was a little more reluctant about the fact that she would be carrying a child with whom she would have no genetic tie. She admitted to being afraid that she would feel as though she were "carrying someone else's baby." But she was desperate to experience pregnancy, and she knew how much Joe wanted a child, so she finally acquiesced.

The first donor that Caroline and Joe selected looked very much like Caroline, with a similar ethnic background. The donor produced only 6 eggs, 4 of which fertilized. Of these, only two reached the 8-cell stage, and were transferred. Unfortunately, Carolyn did not become pregnant. The couple decided to try once more, but this time with a different donor. For this cycle, they selected a woman who looked less like Caroline but whose eggs had been successfully used in a previous cycle with a different patient. Although this donor did not resemble Caroline, she and Joe liked the doctor's description of the donor's personality.

This donor produced nine mature oocytes, seven of which fertilized. Four embryos were frozen at the single cell stage and three were allowed to grow for an additional 48 hours At that time, two embryos grew to the six and eight cell stages and were transferred, whereas the remaining embryo remained at the two cell stage and was subsequently discarded. The couple was very pleased with the fact that they had frozen embryos remaining in reserve just in case pregnancy did not occur in this treatment cycle. After two weeks of anxious waiting, Caroline learned she was pregnant.

When their son, Matthew, was born 9 months later, Caroline and Joe were overjoyed. Caroline admitted that once she had experienced morning sickness, felt the baby kick, seen his image in her sonograms, she had grown to love the feel of him inside her womb. The lack of a genetic tie with her son had become completely irrelevant. The couple never told anyone about having used an egg donor and, to the best of their knowledge, no one in the family suspected that Matthew was conceived using donated eggs.

GESTATIONAL SURROGACY: CARRYING LIFE FOR ANOTHER

Gestational surrogacy is not intended to be a "rent-a-womb" of convenience for privileged women who are not inclined to carry their own babies. Rather, it is the only and last resort for women who have real medical issues that prevent them from carrying a pregnancy to term. Compared to the frequent need for donated eggs, there are relatively few instances in which a woman has good quality oocytes but cannot carry a pregnancy. The most common reasons for surrogacy are cases in which a woman has lost her uterus yet retained her ovaries, because of cervical or uterine cancer or as a result of a life-saving hysterectomy to stop uncontrollable bleeding after childbirth. Even more rarely, a woman who has normal ovaries, is born without a uterus or with an abnormally formed uterus that cannot be surgically corrected. There are also women who have medical conditions like heart disease, or who have had a kidney transplant that are not healthy enough to carry a pregnancy.

In other situations, surrogacy seems to be the only option for certain other women because carrying a pregnancy to term has proved to be impossible because of repetitive late miscarriages occurring between the 16th and 26th week of pregnancy. These cases may have diverse clinical presentations, such as repeated intrauterine fetal demises, premature rupture of the amniotic membranes, or an incompetent uterine cervix. These women have lost their pregnancies every time that they have conceived, despite having received proper medical treatment.

Another group of women habitually have midtrimester pregnancy losses because they have benign uterine conditions such as fibroids (extremely common growths of the uterus) or adenomyosis, (endometriosis found within the muscular walls of the uterus). These conditions interfere with the blood supply between the uterus and the placenta, which provides oxygen to the fetus. Although surgical removal of fibroids often proves successful in preventing future pregnancy losses, there are some instances in which surgical treatment does not prove curative, or is impossible to undertake because of the size or locations of the fibroids. The only curative treatment for adenomyosis is a hysterectomy. Medical treatments for both conditions are temporary and will not help a woman carry a pregnancy to term. The only hope for women with these otherwise untreatable conditions to have their own biological child is with gestational surrogacy.

Having a baby by means of gestational surrogacy is an extremely complex and costly undertaking. Surrogacy, in many states, is illegal except in certain situations in which the gestational carrier is not paid a fee for her services. Furthermore, since the woman who gives birth to the baby is its legal mother, a couple who has a surrogate carry their biologic child must actually adopt their baby after its birth. Such situations could possibly end in a nasty custody fight between the carrier and the biologic parents.

There are many costs involved in gestational surrogacy. Lawyers specializing in reproductive law are needed by all the involved parties. Even if no compensation is paid directly to the gestational carrier (we all know that funds do change hands except in cases where the carrier is a close relative or friend), there are surrogate agency recruitment fees, the cost of the IVF treatment, and the obstetrical and maternity hospital costs. The cost to a couple for having a baby using a gestational carrier could easily range from $50,000 -$100,000. Nevertheless, if this is the only way for a couple to have their own biologic child, I am sure that those who are successfully able to do it find it a miraculous answer to their prayers.

SUMMARY

If deteriorating eggs or a diminished egg supply, or a damaged or absent uterus are keeping you from having a baby, using donated eggs or a gestational carrier may offer you a realistic hope of realizing your dream. Pregnancy rates are high, and when properly coordinated, the procedure itself is relatively easy. The financial and emotional costs associated with these procedures are undoubtedly high, but no one ever said that miracles come without a price!!!

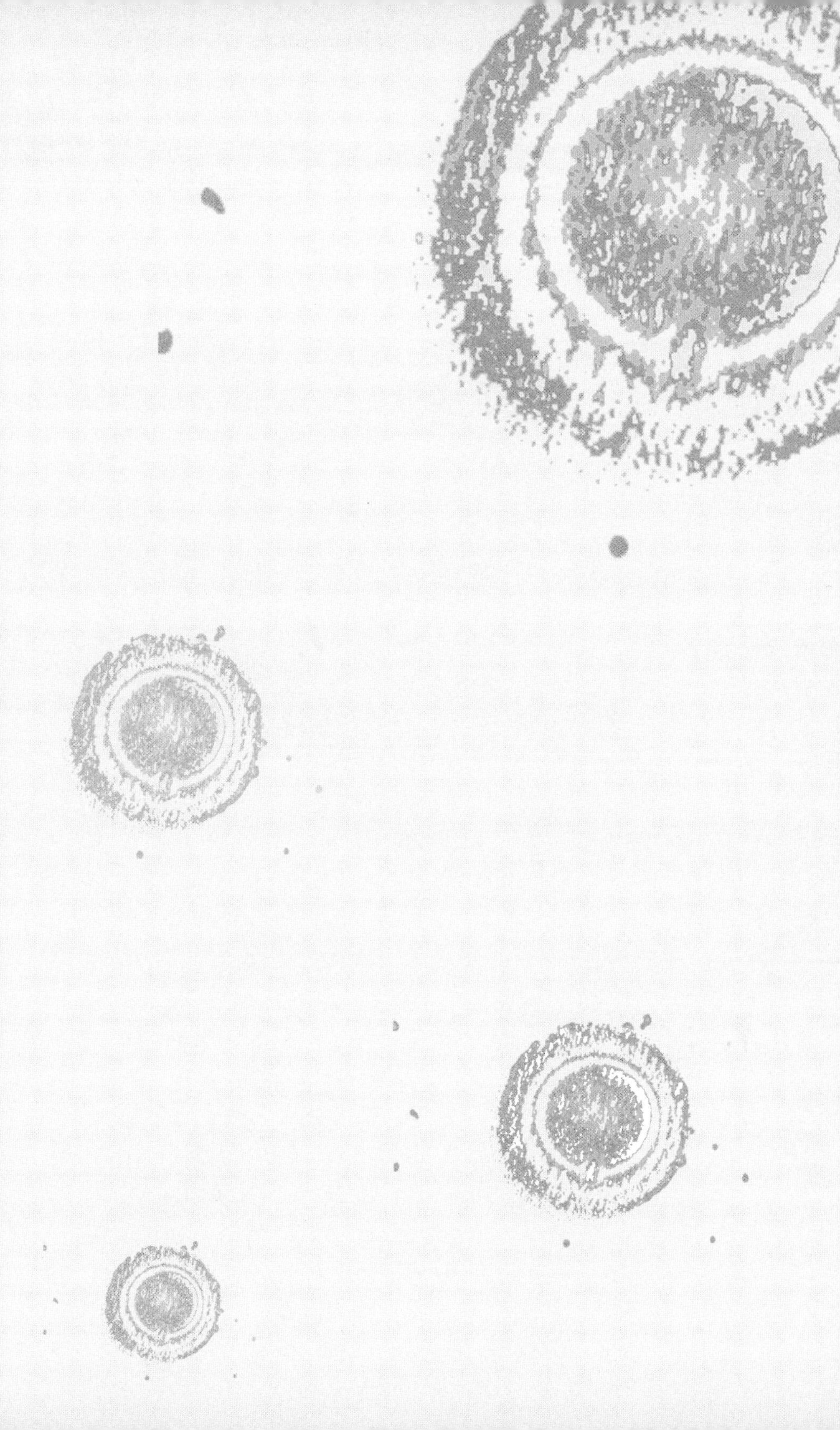

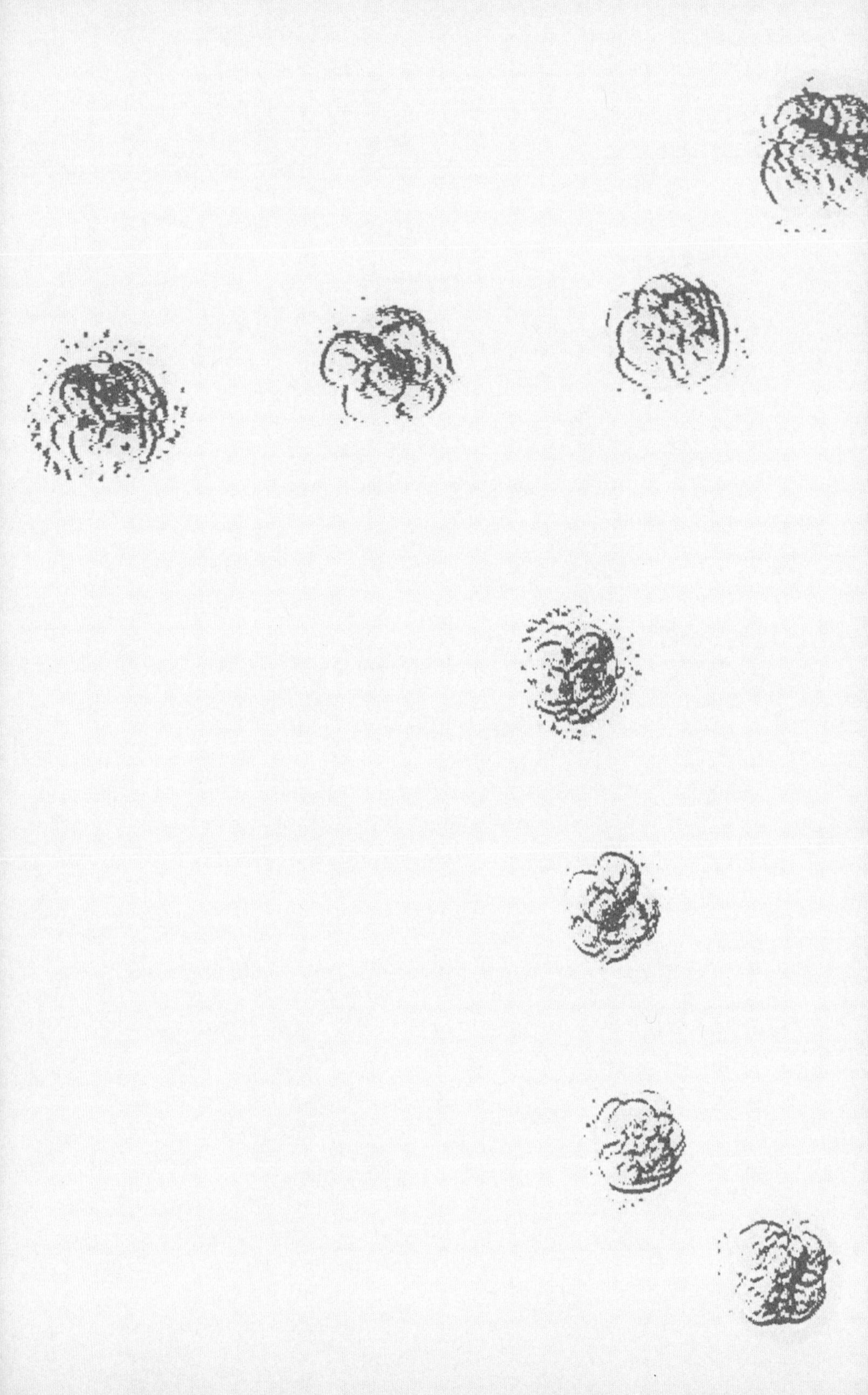

CHAPTER 12

PREIMPLANTATION GENETIC DIAGNOSIS:

Things You Must Know About Genetics To Better Understand Infertility

Preimplantation Genetic Diagnosis (PGD) is a procedure that is employed to analyze certain aspects of the chromosomal content of individual embryos. For example, PGD is an extremely reliable method for determining the sex of an embryo as it can identify an X or a Y chromosome without error. A clinical example of medically indicated sex selection using PGD is the case in which a couple has a family history of hemophilia, which is a genetic disease that affects only males. IVF with PGD could be employed to enable only the transfer of female embryos, which would be free of this serious disease.

PGD is also very useful for determining if an embryo is affected with certain types of the more common genetic abnormalities such as Down's syndrome, in which there is an extra chromosome #21. For patients at a high risk for having a Down's syndrome baby and who are not able to terminate such a pregnancy because of their religious or ethical beliefs, PGD is able to ensure that any embryo transferred will not be affected with Down's syndrome if it implants and develops into a viable pregnancy. In fact, there are literally hundreds of very rare genetic diseases that can be tested for at the embryonic level, as long as the chromosomal location of the abnormal gene is known. The presence of a specific genetic abnormality in the family must be known in advance so that special preparations can be made to test for that particular genetically transmitted disease. There is currently no test available that can test for all genetic diseases in a single embryo, nor can any embryo be tested to insure that it is perfectly healthy. That crucial task is left to Mother Nature, who will inevitably prevent an unhealthy embryo from implanting or reaching the point that it is born alive.

As you have read in Chapter 1, it is impossible to look at an embryo and tell whether it has a normal number of chromosomes or is aneuploidic or otherwise genetically abnormal. The ability to be able to count the number of chromosome strands in each embryo would ensure that only embryos having the normal complement of 23 chromosome pairs would be selected for transfer. If aneuploidy were the only genetic factor involved in the development of a healthy baby, transferring only embryos with a normal number of chromosomes should result in a 100% pregnancy rate per embryo transfer. Obviously this is not the case, since the pregnancy rate obtained after the transfer of embryos judged to be of normal chromosome number is actually below 50%.

Since embryos thought to have a normal number of chromosome strands are not guaranteed to possess the degree of genetic perfection that is required to produce a viable pregnancy, there must be deeper levels of genetic complexities involved. In fact, chromosomal number may only be the most superficial layer of factors that permit the development of a normal, healthy baby. The deeper genetic layers actually involve the individual genes themselves, located on a specific site on each chromosome strand. As many as 1,000-2,000 individual gene sites may be found on a single chromosomal strand. These gene sites must be in perfect alignment with each other when the male and female chromosome strands unite at the time of fertilization. If the chromosomes do not align themselves perfectly with each other, "lethal genes" may cause the embryo to form in such a way that is not compatible with life. There is also another genetic phenomenon known as translocation, in which portions of matching chromosome strands will be interchanged with each other. Some instances of translocation may not affect the health of the embryo, while others prove lethal. These are the most probable reasons that an embryo with a normal number of chromosomes will either fail to implant or create a pregnancy that will ultimately end in miscarriage. Based upon the potential for genetic errors occurring during the process of fertilization, such as the ones mentioned previously, even if an embryo grows at a normal rate and appears to be completely normal when examined under a microscope, it is statistically more likely than not to be genetically abnormal, especially if it is derived from the eggs of a woman who is over the age of 35.

PGD: THE PROCEDURE

PGD is an invasive procedure performed for genetic analysis. In PGD, one or two cells are microsurgically removed robotically from an 8-cell embryo on the third day of its life. Although the removal of 12-25% of the cellular elements of an embryo may seem a bit radical, it usually does not have an adverse effect the future growth and development of an embryo. The reason for this is that, theoretically, all the cells that comprise an embryo have identical genetic material, so that the removed cells are quickly replaced by other cells that are their "clones," Although it rarely happens, the insertion of a microscopic needle into an embryo could potentially destroy an embryo.

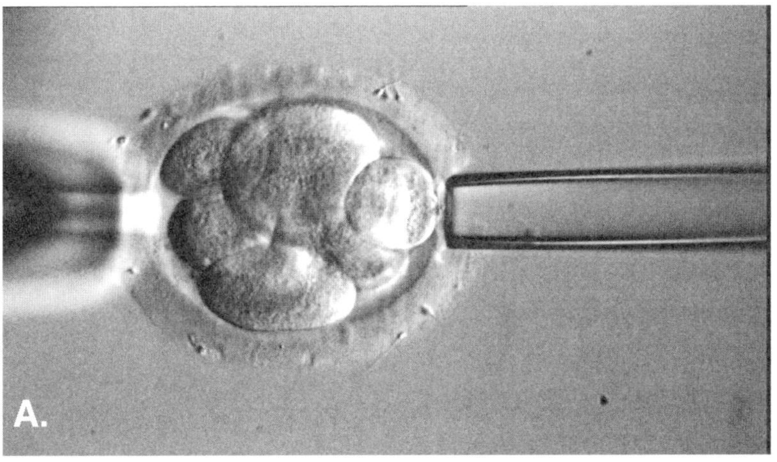

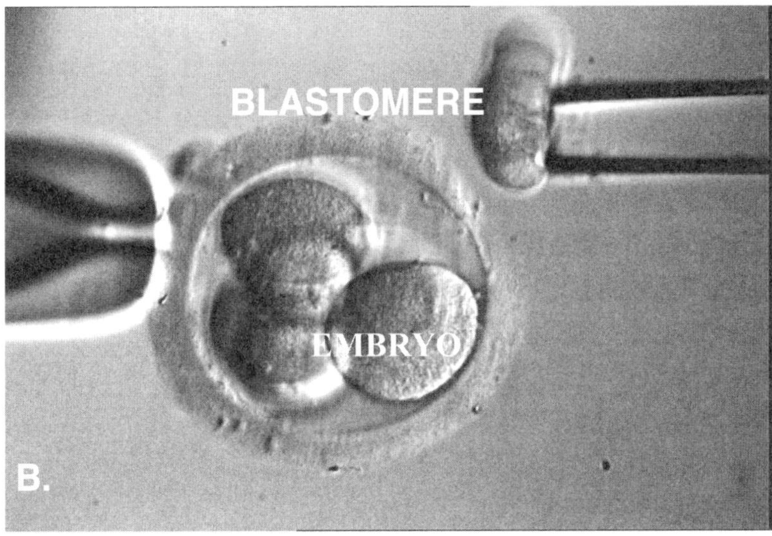

Fig. 1. A. ***Embryo biopsy for PGD.***
B. ***Embryonic cell (blastomere) removed from the embryo, which will be analyzed genetically.***

Once the cell, called a blastomere, is microscopically removed from the embryo, it is fixed to a special slide and is then submitted by express courier to a very specialized laboratory that exclusively performs genetic testing on embryos.

This laboratory will return the results for each embryo biopsied within 24 hours, so that the transfer of genetically optimal embryos can be done on day 5 when they have reached the blastocyst stage. The embryos found to have either too many or too few chromosomes are discarded, since they will not result in a normal pregnancy.

PGD testing is costly; it adds another $3,500 – $5,000 to the basic price of an IVF procedure. Further increasing the cost of the process is that all embryos biopsied for PGD must be fertilized by ICSI so that no other sperm cells, which contain extraneous chromosomal strands, are bound to the outside of the embryo. This adds another $1,000-$2500 to the procedure. Depending upon the IVF center and its location, an IVF cycle with PGD could cost between $12,000 and $16,000, exclusive of medications, anesthesia, and facility fees. Often, PGD solely for the purpose of diagnosing aneuploidy is not covered by insurance. If PGD is covered by insurance, it is only in clinical situations when it is used to reduce the risk of transmission of a genetic disease or for a reduction of the risk of miscarriage in a woman who has had more than three consecutive "misses." The reason that PGD is so costly is that the biopsy of an embryo is a microscopic robotic surgical procedure requiring very expensive equipment and is performed by a highly skilled (and highly paid) embryologist. The other component of the cost is the laboratory testing itself, which also requires extremely expensive equipment, reagents and highly trained personnel.

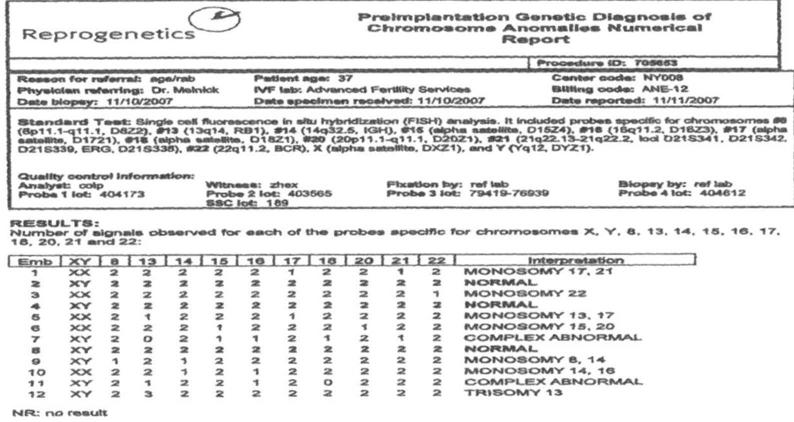

Reprogenetics

Preimplantation Genetic Diagnosis of Chromosome Anomalies Numerical Report

Procedure ID: 705653

Reason for referral: age/rab | Patient age: 37 | Center code: NY008
Physician referring: Dr. Melnick | IVF lab: Advanced Fertility Services | Billing code: ANE-12
Date biopsy: 11/10/2007 | Date specimen received: 11/10/2007 | Date reported: 11/11/2007

Standard Test: Single cell fluorescence in situ hybridization (FISH) analysis. It included probes specific for chromosomes #8 (8p11.1-q11.1, D8Z2), #13 (13q14, RB1), #14 (14q32.5, IGH), #15 (alpha satellite, D15Z4), #16 (16q11.2, D16Z3), #17 (alpha satellite, D17Z1), #18 (alpha satellite, D18Z1), #20 (20p11.1-q11.1, D20Z1), #21 (21q22.13-21q22.2, loci D21S341, D21S342, D21S339, ERG, D21S338), #22 (22q11.2, BCR), X (alpha satellite, DXZ1), and Y (Yq12, DYZ1).

Quality control information:
Analyst: colp | Witness: zhex | Fixation by: ref lab | Biopsy by: ref lab
Probe 1 lot: 404173 | Probe 2 lot: 403565 | Probe 3 lot: 79419-76939 | Probe 4 lot: 404612
SSC lot: 189

RESULTS:
Number of signals observed for each of the probes specific for chromosomes X, Y, 8, 13, 14, 15, 16, 17, 18, 20, 21 and 22:

Emb	XY	8	13	14	15	16	17	18	20	21	22	Interpretation
1	XX	2	2	2	2	2	1	2	2	1	2	MONOSOMY 17, 21
2	XY	2	2	2	2	2	2	2	2	2	2	NORMAL
3	XX	2	2	2	2	2	2	2	2	2	1	MONOSOMY 22
4	XY	2	2	2	2	2	2	2	2	2	2	NORMAL
5	XX	2	1	2	2	2	1	2	2	2	2	MONOSOMY 13, 17
6	XX	2	2	2	1	2	2	2	1	2	2	MONOSOMY 15, 20
7	XY	2	0	2	1	1	2	1	2	1	2	COMPLEX ABNORMAL
8	XY	2	2	2	2	2	2	2	2	2	2	NORMAL
9	XY	1	2	1	2	2	2	2	2	2	2	MONOSOMY 8, 14
10	XX	2	2	1	2	1	2	2	2	2	2	MONOSOMY 14, 16
11	XY	2	1	2	2	1	2	0	2	2	2	COMPLEX ABNORMAL
12	XY	2	3	2	2	2	2	2	2	2	2	TRISOMY 13

NR: no result

Fig. 2. ***PGD report of the analysis of 12 chromosomes in 12 different embryos. Note that only 3 out of 12 embryos were genetically normal. These three embryos were transferred and resulted in a viable twin pregnancy.***

RESULTS:
Number of signals observed for each of the probes specific for chromosomes X, Y, 8, 13, 14, 15, 16, 17, 18, 20, 21 and 22:

Emb	XY	8	13	14	15	16	17	18	20	21	22	INTERPRETATION
1	XY	2	2	2	2	2	3	1	2	2	2	MONOSOMY 18, TRISOMY 17
2	XO	2	3	1	2	1	2	1	1	2	1	COMPLEX ABNORMAL
3	XX	1	1	2	2	3	1	2	1	1	2	COMPLEX ABNORMAL
4	XY	2	2	2	2	2	2	2	2	2	2	NORMAL

Fig. 3. ***PGD report from a young woman who has had several previous miscarriages. Note that only 1 out of 4 of the embryos was genetically normal. Unfortunately, the transfer of that embryo did not produce a pregnancy.***

A potentially greater issue is that the PGD testing of embryonic cells can be inherently inaccurate, even though all aspects of the laboratory procedure are done perfectly. The first inherent potential inaccuracy results from the fact that only a maximum of 12 chromosome pairs can be tested, not all 23. The primary reason for this is that there is simply not enough time to test all 23 pairs. Testing must be completed during the fourth day of laboratory culture, so that results are available by the time that the embryos reach the blastocyst stage on the fifth day of growth. Embryos must be transferred into the uterus before the sixth day, at which time the embryos "hatch" out of their protective shell. The twelve chromosome pairs that are tested are the ones that were most frequently found to be abnormal when genetic analysis of miscarried fetal tissue was performed. Although the 12 chromosome pairs tested are the ones most commonly involved in embryonic genetic abnormalities, it is quite possible to have extra strands of chromosomes that are not included in the group that is routinely tested. Therefore, an embryo that is determined to be normal by PGD testing could actually be abnormal because its abnormality involves a chromosome pair that is not routinely tested. This is one of the principle reasons that the transfer of embryos deemed to be genetically normal by PGD is not 100% successful. In fact, the pregnancy rate is considerably less than 50%, even when one or two embryos judged to be normal by PGD are transferred into the uterus.

There have also been reports of instances when embryos declared to be abnormal by PGD have actually produced healthy babies. This has occurred in rare instances in which a couple elected to transfer an embryo missing only one strand of chromosomal material, when none of their other embryos were found to be "normal." How could this have possibly occurred? It seems that PGD may not always be accurate when the chromosome complement of an embryo is missing one strand. In cases in which one of the twelve chromosome pairs tested is found to have only one strand, a condition called monosomy occurs. Of course, when one chromosome strand is missing, it would seem obvious that the embryo is abnormal and should not be transferred back into the uterus. It seems that PGD, on certain rare occasions, may fail to identify a chromosome strand, so an otherwise normal embryo may be erroneously called monosomic. Fairly recent developments in the laboratory technique for PGD enable the further evaluation of cells that have monosomic, indeterminate or otherwise questionable readings so as to prevent genetically normal embryos from being labeled as abnormal and discarded. However, some experts in this field are now recommending the routine transfer of monosomic embryos, since true monosomic (except monosomic embryos with a single X or 21 chromosome) never develop into blastocysts. Since there is documented case precedence, I would suggest that monosomic embryos could be transferred, but whenever they are, chorionic villus sampling or amniocentesis should be performed if miscarriage does not occur during the first ten weeks of gestation. Again, I believe that the process of natural selection will eliminate truly unhealthy embryos with more precision than the most sophisticated laboratory tests.

In addition to the limitation in the number of chromosomes that are tested, there is another very subtle pitfall that may affect the diagnostic accuracy of PGD. As I mentioned earlier in this chapter, it is assumed that all the blastomeres in a particular embryo are genetically identical. According to the established laws of genetics, all the cells in an individual's body (with the exception of egg and sperm cells, each of which has a unique genetic contribution from one of our ancestors) should have exactly the same genetic composition. Because their genetic composition should theoretically be identical, when two cells from an embryo are tested with PGD, identical results -whether normal or abnormal- should be obtained. Unfortunately, this is not always the case. It seems that the laws of genetics are not quite as universal as would be believed. Occasionally, an embryo somehow acquires an extra cell line so that it contains blastomeres that have two distinctly different genetic patterns—as if there were fraternal twins residing in a single embryo. This is a phenomenon known as genetic chimerism. The original Chimera was a mythological creature made up of parts of different animals- the head of a lion, the body of a goat and the tail of a dragon. A chimeric embryo, therefore, has two distinct cell populations which could seriously interfere with the accuracy of PGD, since testing may give a result based upon only one cell line. Even if two blastomeres are tested, the presence of a second cell line can still be missed. Technically, embryonic chimerism is more correctly referred to as genetic mosaicism, since the two cell lines result from genetic events within a single embryo, rather than from the fusion of two embryos. Nevertheless, studies exist showing that a surprisingly high number of day three embryos, at the 8 cell stage, were found to have some degree of mosaicism. The most incredible finding was that the mosaicism disappears in the vast majority of cases by the time the embryo reaches the blastocyst stage. It is as if the embryo has the ability to heal itself if it is ultimately destined to be healthy enough to form a viable pregnancy! Although mosaicism can be found in a significant percentage of the healthy population, its presence in an individual is never detected unless they are involved in a paternity case or in organ donation situation for a sibling or a child, which requires DNA testing.

There was a fascinating example of genetic chimerism in a case in which DNA test results performed for a child custody issue indicated that a child's documented birth mother, the woman who carried him in her womb for nine months, was not its "real" genetic mother. Her DNA did not match that of her own child. How could this be possible? This poor woman was tortured by the legal system until someone guessed that she was a genetic chimera. To prove that she was the child's mother, cells from many different tissues in her body were tested. While her white blood cells, which are the usual cells tested for DNA analysis, were completely different from her child's', cells from other tissues in her body, like her ovary, thyroid and kidney (which all required biopsy to test), matched the child perfectly.

WHERE PGD MAY HELP

Although it has certain inherent problems, PGD may be appropriate for use in two frequently occurring clinical settings. The first is the situation in which a woman has multiple pregnancy losses before the tenth week of pregnancy. These pregnancy losses are almost always caused by genetic factors, with abnormal chromosome numbers often found in the miscarried fetal tissue. A miscarriage is devastating for any couple, but it is even more so for those who have had difficulty in conceiving. After having one miscarriage, a couple will naturally experience incredibly high levels of anxiety with their next conception. From the moment of the first positive pregnancy test, the couple finds themselves "holding their breath" until they pass out of the danger zone for pregnancy loss. PGD is often utilized to alleviate a great deal of the angst that these couples must endure.

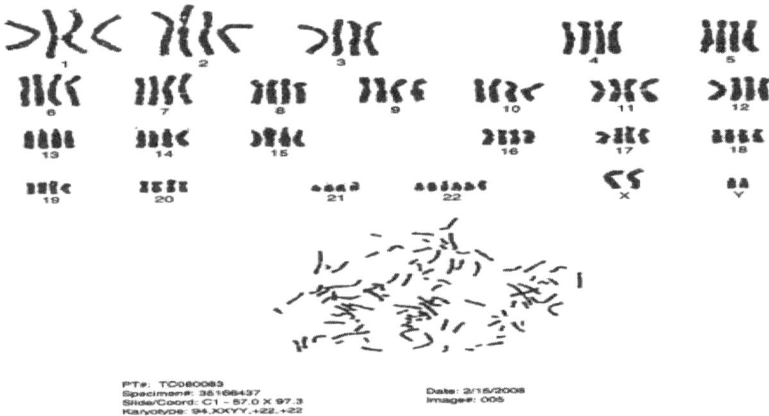

Fig. 4. ***This is the genetic analysis of tissue from a miscarried pregnancy. Note that there are double the normal number of chromosomes. There is also an extra chromosome number 22. This is a classical example of aneuploidy.***

By eliminating aneuploid embryos and transferring only embryos with the normal complement of 46 chromosomes, it would seem that the chance of a miscarriage caused by aneuploidy should be significantly reduced and the live birth rate be increased. Unfortunately, reality is not always logical. Recent data from certain European fertility centers suggest that PGD testing of embryos for aneuploidy may not increase the live birth rate in couples who have had a previous high incidence of miscarriage in the group of patients that they studied. This is contrary to data from PGD laboratories in the U.S, which demonstrated that PGD testing significantly increased the live birth rate in those patients with a history of prior recurrent early pregnancy loss. Currently, there is a rather vigorous ongoing debate between the American and European researchers as to whether PGD is beneficial in this capacity. The two groups of scientists continue to do battle over this issue; thus far, there is no clear victor.

In the United States, most fertility specialists offer PGD to couples who are prone to frequent early miscarriages. I think that this use of PGD is quite legitimate, especially for those couples who have become severely depressed and cannot emotionally deal with the possibility of having another miscarriage. Utilizing PGD gives couples a sense of control of their reproductive destiny in the sense that the implantation of a genetically abnormal embryo, which will inevitably miscarry, cannot be prevented if conception happens naturally. However, couples should understand that when using PGD to eliminate aneuploidic embryos there is always the possibility that all the embryos tested will be abnormal and none will be transferred. They must also remember that even if an embryo is found to be normal with PGD testing, it may not grow to reach the blastocyst stage, and hence cannot be transferred. Moreover, a blastocyst that is considered normal by PGD evaluation will implant significantly less than 50% of the time. Pregnancy after PGD is not guaranteed. The best way to summarize the advantage of PGD is that it can prevent miscarriage by eliminating aneuploid embryos but it cannot guarantee that conception will occur after the transfer of embryos determined to be normal after PGD testing.

On the other hand, my belief in nature and natural selection, as well as my clinical experiences prior to the days of IVF and PGD, does not allow me to recommend PGD for all couples who have endured multiple pregnancy losses. Over the years, I have seen a number of patients who have had normal pregnancies after as many as seven early first trimester miscarriages. I share such clinical experiences with couples who have had normal genetic testing themselves (karyotype analysis) and who do not have a female age factor. If they can conceive easily, they could elect to continue to try conceiving naturally and still have a realistic chance that that a normal pregnancy will eventually be achieved. Likewise, in women over age 35, in whom miscarriage is most likely caused by aneuploidy, I recommend that they trust in nature to produce a healthy pregnancy, with the understanding that there is a chance that a normal pregnancy may not be possible for them under any circumstances as a result of their age and the genetic quality of their eggs.

I would like to share with you my recollection of a lecture on the treatment of miscarriage that I heard as a medical student in 1968. As I recall, the professor described a study which was performed to compare the common treatment modalities used at that time: complete bed rest, "hormone injections" (progesterone or a synthetic estrogen) or frequent visits to the doctor. The women who visited their doctors most frequently, with no other treatments other than an internal examination to verify that the uterus was growing, had the highest rate of live births. Despite the fact that clinical studies in those days were not nearly as scientifically rigorous as the ones published today, I have always believed that frequent medical follow up visits are extremely beneficial to patients' general sense of well being. The earliest part of a pregnancy is both a time of great joy and great anxiety. It is a critical time for emotional support, best supplied by their doctor. Combined with the information supplied by sonographic examinations, a couple can see the actual state of their pregnancy on a weekly basis. If the pregnancy is developing well, they receive realistic reassurance and their level of stress is kept low. Should a problem be seen, there is time for the couple to prepare themselves emotionally for the loss of the pregnancy. In such cases, the pregnancy can be terminated at an early stage, before the couple has too much emotional investment in it.

The other possible use for PGD is in cases of implantation failure in young women who would, on the surface, appear to be ideal candidates for IVF and yet do not achieve conception despite the production of many perfectly formed embryos during the course of multiple IVF cycles. Most often, these patients fall within two diagnostic categories: unexplained infertility and polycystic ovarian syndrome. Although the patients these groups are quite different in many respects, they share common ground in that they have a large ovarian reserve of oocytes, they are high responders to fertility medications in terms of egg production and have relatively low pregnancy rates. Although they seem to be excellent responders to IVF treatment, their pregnancy rates are far below those of women requiring IVF as a result of blocked Fallopian tubes or a male factor.

The reduction of pregnancy rates in these women is most often due to a high rate of genetic imperfections in the embryos themselves. It is rarely due to a problem with uterine receptivity unless there are demonstrable abnormalities in the uterus, such as poor endometrial development, fibroids or adenomyosis (endometriosis inside the walls of the uterus). The use of PGD testing to sort out genetically abnormal embryos should help pregnancy rates by identifying and eliminating abnormal embryos while enabling the transfer and cryopreservation of only the best embryos. PGD testing is also of value in helping couples get an understanding of the genetic basis of their infertility, since many couples erroneously blame themselves for their failure to conceive. I believe that PGD has potential value in this regard. But when embryos found to be normal with PGD testing, are transferred repeatedly and pregnancy still does not occur, the couple is really in a more difficult position than they had been previously. Their infertility is due to either genetic factors in the embryo that are not detectable by ordinary means or there exists a uterine factor that cannot be diagnosed or treated. Unfortunately, such cases of implantation failure which elude diagnosis and treatment are encountered. Adoption, donor oocytes or a gestational carrier are all options that can be considered in those cases. Yet, an interesting statistic comes to mind: 3% of couples who have longstanding unexplained infertility and who adopt a baby will eventually conceive on their own. Does this mean that such couples have become more "relaxed" and, as such, are able to conceive? Or did a genetically perfect egg and sperm finally meet, joining their chromosomes in such a way that a perfect embryo is formed which is capable of developing into a viable pregnancy? The answers to these questions can never really be known, but merely raise more questions that are, themselves, entirely unanswerable.

SUMMARY

After reading this chapter, it can easily be seen just how far the current state of preimplantation genetic diagnosis is from perfection. In the future, we can only hope for the perfect test of embryonic quality which would enable the transfer of a single embryo with a normal complement of 23 chromosome pairs which are in perfect alignment and without translocations. Of course the test must be able to be produce results rapidly, so that the transfer can be performed prior to the sixth day of embryonic life, when the embryo hatches. There is currently available a method that is available which can detect all 23 chromosome pairs, called Comparative Genomic Hybridization.

This technology shows some promise, but it requires three weeks to produce results, so any embryos tested must be cryopreserved and transferred at a later date if found to be genetically normal. Although it seems that geneticists are heading in the right direction, the process of fertilization and embryo development is so complex that I seriously doubt that the day will ever come that geneticists will have the ability to select a genetically perfect embryo that has an implantation rate of 100%. It seems to me that only nature and natural selection will ever have this amazing capability.

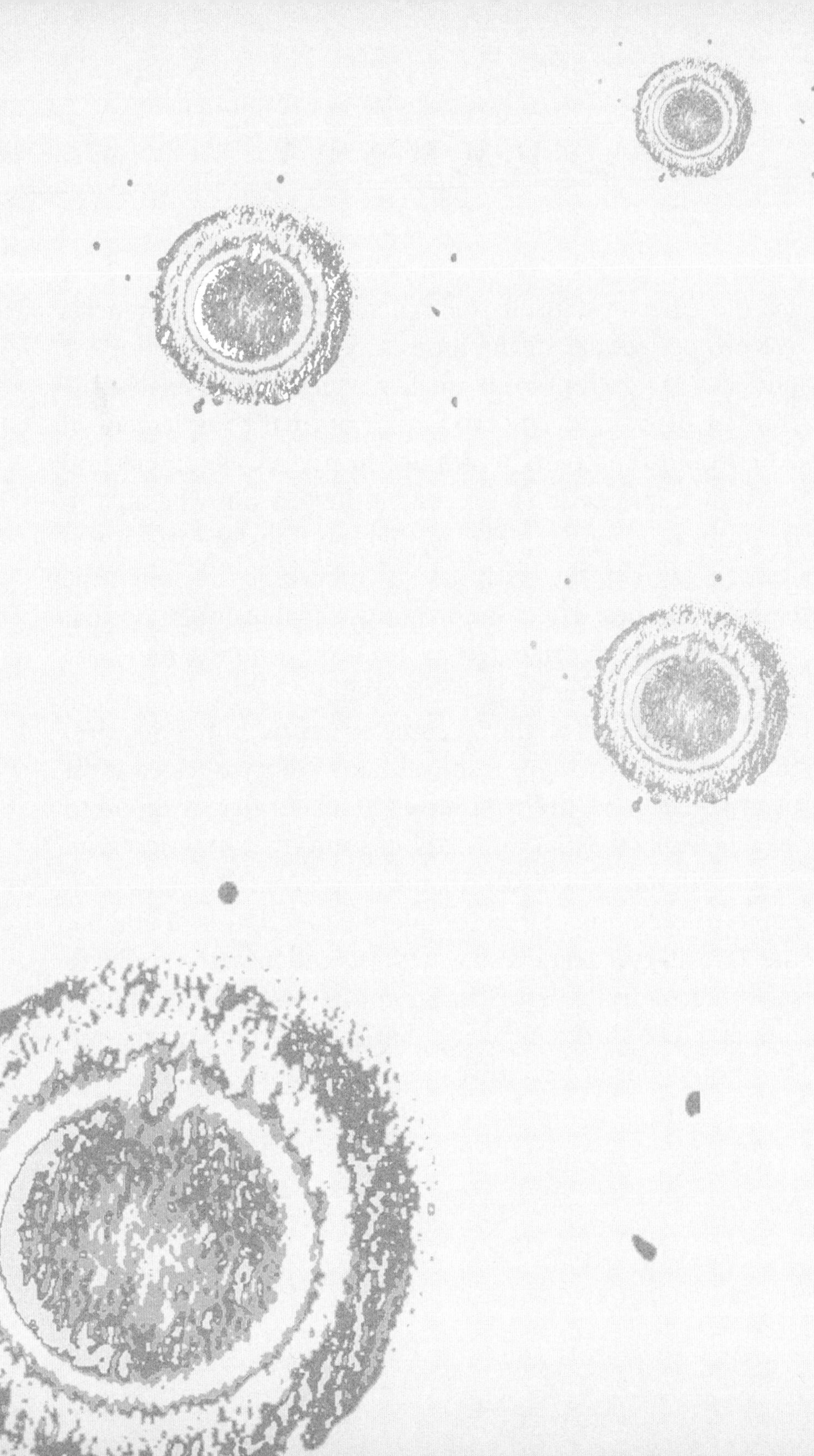

CHAPTER 13

BEGINNING YOUR JOURNEY:

Important Considerations

In *The Pregnancy Prescription,* I have described a pathway to help couples understand the various diagnostic and treatment options that are currently available to help them achieve their goal of having a baby. Hopefully, the preceeding chapters will have provided an in-depth factual basis that will be of assistance in making the proper choices in their quest for conception.

This journey begins with the choice of an infertility specialist or IVF center. This decision is an extremely important one, as it will ultimately determine the course that a couple's treatment will follow. Moreover, it will determine the quality of a couple's experience, which is so critical to the outcome. If the couple's experiences during the process of infertility treatment are generally pleasant and not too stressful, they will be more likely to have a better chance of persevering until a positive outcome is obtained. On the other hand, should their experiences be overly stressful and unpleasant, they may be unable to "hang in there" long enough for the statistical odds inherent in the process of conception to work in their favor. Therefore, I would like to close this book by offering some thoughts, observations and some "plain old-fashioned" common sense advice that will aid you in the selection process.

CHOOSING A DOCTOR

Most couples choose a fertility specialist or clinic based on a recommendation from a friend or a physician, from their insurance carrier's list of providers or from researching websites on the Internet. The recommendation of an individual who has actually received treatment from a certain specialist or clinic is a reliable source of referral. Whether that individual was able to conceive or not, he or she may be a source of relevant information that could be useful in helping to shape a proper decision. Unfortunately, many couples are hesitant to reveal that they had infertility problems and are therefore unwilling to share their experiences and information. Other individuals are afraid to make a recommendation, fearing that the referral may not work out well. Although a recommendation based on personal experience is an excellent place to start the search for fertility treatment, these recommendations—whether made by a friend or a physician—may have some element of bias.

The most important thing to keep in mind is that if you do not have a positive feeling about a fertility specialist after your initial consultation, you should trust your instincts and seek care elsewhere. This is true regardless of the source of your original referral. Even if the person who made the recommendation conceived under the care of this doctor and firmly believes that he or she is a "miracle worker," you must be comfortable with the physician's manner and the way in which you are treated in his or her clinic; do not start treatment if your "inner voice" expresses reservations.

In addition to assessing your personal reaction to the physician, you should understand their approach to infertility treatments in general, as well as their specific approach to your unique clinical situation. During your initial consultation, a physician should not only obtain a relevant medical history but also map out a game plan that spells out the schedule of diagnostic tests and the nature of the possible treatment options. There should also be ample time for you to ask questions and express any concerns or anxieties that you might have. Irrespective of a doctor's reputation or credentials, if he or she seems rushed, distracted or otherwise inattentive, you may rest assured that they will not give you the personalized care that you require. Nearly all practitioners in the field today have similar training and credentials—that is, they are board certified by the American College of Obstetricians and Gynecologists. Most are also "success-oriented" and employ the approach advocated in the first volume of *The Pregnancy Prescription,* written nearly ten years ago. If you find that a doctor is proposing a diagnostically oriented approach to your infertility problem, insisting upon a battery of tests, you should immediately head for the hills! You should also avoid celebrity doctors that appear frequently in the media, as media coverage doesn't guarantee that the physician is a uniquely talented practitioner or an especially compassionate caregiver.

CHOOSING AN IVF CLINIC

It is important to understand that today, compared with ten years ago, most IVF clinics are essentially equal thanks to the high level of regulatory compliance required to offer fertility services. Fertility clinics must be licensed and are inspected on a regular basis by both state and federal regulatory agencies. Every clinic that is registered with the Society of Reproductive Medicine (S.A.R.T.) must adhere to the same high standard of practice. Having membership in S.A.R.T. and submitting their data to the Center for Disease Control (C.D.C.) means that a fertility center is a legitimate provider of IVF services. If a center is not listed, I would be hesitant to engage its services.

Today, all IVF clinics employ similar ovarian stimulation protocols, as well as egg retrieval and embryo transfer procedures. In addition, all IVF laboratories employ similar embryo culture media, equipment and techniques. Established IVF centers are required to be staffed with experienced embryologists that have proven their capabilities in embryo culture, ICSI and other laboratory techniques that have resulted in a significant number of clinical pregnancies. In essence, you as a patient and a consumer should feel comfortable that you are protected from fly by night clinics, which may still operate in other areas of clinical practice such as cosmetic surgery and other related aesthetic services.

A significant difference that does exist among IVF clinics is the populations of patients that they treat. Patient populations have a large impact on a clinic's rate of live births, which must be reported to both S.A.R.T. and the C.D.C. For example, if an IVF clinic treats a population of patients with a large number of male factor patients (whose female partners usually have good egg quality), the rate of clinical pregnancies will be higher than one with a patient population that has a larger proportion of patients with unexplained infertility, endometriosis or polycystic ovarian syndrome. Patients in these diagnostic categories generally take more treatment cycles to conceive as a result of diminished egg quality associated with these conditions. It is important to understand that statistics can only give the general probability of conception within a broad diagnostic range of large numbers of patients of a certain age group.

Differences in success rates among clinics may be due to the prognosis of the patients that are treated by the clinic. For instance, a clinic could "stack the deck" by being overly selective in terms of the patients it treats with IVF. Patients in the diagnostic categories with the highest predicted pregnancy rates (for example, those in which the woman has the highest ovarian reserve and the lowest FSH levels) would be encouraged to undergo treatment with IVF while patients with a poorer prognostic outlook (for example, women with low ovarian reserve and relatively high FSH levels for their age) may be discouraged from trying IVF and would instead be advised to go directly to a donor egg program or be treated with repetitive cycles of controlled ovarian hyperstimulation and IUI. Restricting IVF treatment to patients with optimal prognoses in this way will give a clinic the highest live birth rates. Alternatively, clinics serving patient populations with a higher incidence of low ovarian reserve, endometriosis and unexplained infertility will have significantly lower live birth rates, despite offering medical services of the highest quality. In addition, a fertility clinic may have excellent clinical pregnancy rates yet, due to an unusually high rate of pregnancy loss through miscarriage and obstetrical complications, have a relatively low live birth rate.

As stated in the preface to the C.D.C.'s annual report, the IVF live birth rate is not a valid basis for making a comparison among clinics. The truth is, such statistics have little relevance to an individual couple, since each is a unique entity that is not exactly comparable to any other couple in the same group. Therefore, statistical probabilities cannot be used to predict a couple's chance of conception on a given IVF cycle. Getting pregnant is not a numbers game, so a couple's chance of becoming pregnant by going to a clinic with a higher percentage of live births is not necessarily better than if they seek treatment at a facility that has a lower success rate.

Finally, a fertility clinic's data is frequently out of date by the time these data are published by the C.D.C.. The data lag occurs because it takes nine months after the last conception of the calendar year for the final birth to be documented. For example, the last IVF conception of 2007, in December, will not deliver until mid-September 2008. The C.D.C. cannot make the 2007 pregnancy data available to the public until the spring of 2009. Of course, such information is quite out of date and is of limited relevance.

Although the S.A.R.T. and C.D.C data is somewhat limited in its value for selecting an IVF clinic, the information submitted by participating clinics is very accurate. When an IVF clinic submits its data to S.A.R.T and the C.D.C, it is via a complex Internet program that makes the manipulation of data impossible. In addition, clinics that are part of S.A.R.T. are subject to unannounced audits of their medical records to verify the accuracy of the data that they have submitted. There are serious consequences for submitting inflated data, including—but not limited to—large fines and loss of licensure. If an IVF clinic does not report its success rates to SART and the CDC, I would question its' success rates, since such their data is not verifiable.

HOW SHOULD YOU CHOOSE?

If most infertility specialists have equal training and most IVF center laboratories function in much the same way, what are the key factors that a couple should consider when choosing an infertility treatment program?

From speaking with many patients about their past experiences with fertility therapy, I've found virtually all seek is to be treated by a physician with whom they can have some sort of personal rapport. This connection is commonly referred to as the doctor-patient relationship, and it is an essential part of any patient's therapeutic experience. In other words, a physician must address a patient's emotional issues at the same time that he or she renders medical treatment. This is especially true in reproductive medicine, since virtually all patients find themselves on a monthly emotional rollercoaster ride as they undergo treatment. Patients typically experience varying degrees of anxiety, depression and frustration. The emotional turmoil that patients experience is intensified by the high levels of estrogen and progesterone that are produced by the stimulation of multiple follicles. Therefore, it is vital that fertility specialists address their patients' psychological issues at the same time that they stimulate their ovaries and collect their eggs.

In order to meet their patients' needs in a satisfactory manner, reproductive endocrinologists must take the time to personally communicate with their patients, provide them with an opportunity to express their feelings and give them whatever emotional support that they might need. For example, by taking the time to listen as a patient describes her recent feelings of increased nervousness and depression, a doctor has the opportunity to explain that her symptoms are the result of the high levels of hormones that typically accompany fertility drug treatment. The information provided by the doctor will offer genuine reassurance to the woman.

In addition, when a patient has a strong relationship with a doctor, treatment cycles will be considerably less stressful. When stress levels are high, a patient's energies are depleted and her ability to persevere with treatment is greatly reduced. As you are well aware, most couples require multiple treatment cycles to either become pregnant or to come to the point of resolution of their infertility. Wouldn't it be a pity if a couple who had an excellent chance for conception became so emotionally traumatized by their first IVF experience that they were unable to continue treatment? If they had just been able to persevere with one or more IVF attempts, it is likely that they would have had a baby.

The main message is that the quality of the doctor-patient relationship is the major factor that shapes a couple's treatment experience. For example, if a couple receives treatment in a clinic with a large staff of physicians who work on a rotating basis, the chance of seeing one doctor on a regular basis is nonexistent. Although such an arrangement may be efficient for providing excellent medical treatment to large numbers of patients, it does not allow the formation of a connection between doctor and patient. In such a clinical setting, the doctors may communicate with their patients primarily through nurses and medical assistants. Although a clinic's nursing staff does offer support and guidance, there is really no substitute for an available and caring physician.

Likewise, most patients appreciate an office environment that is friendly and comfortable. When a clinic offers a "take a number and stand in line" experience, the medical treatment offered can be of excellent quality yet the therapeutic experience turns many couples off. If a treatment facility's culture emphasizes statistics and efficiency over sensitivity to the emotional needs of its patients, couples should seriously consider moving to a facility that offers a more emotionally supportive environment. By making such a change, a couple's chances for conception will not be compromised while at the same time the quality of their therapeutic experience will be greatly enhanced.

THE BOTTOM LINE

Advanced reproductive technology is based entirely on well-established scientific principles and laboratory techniques. There are no superstars or miracle workers, and a doctor's skill and a laboratory's proficiency can only make a limited contribution to the process of successful conception. Nature and natural selection, which are entirely beyond human control, are the ultimate determinants of whether a treatment cycle will be successful. Therefore, it is of great importance that couples who require assistance with conception understand these realities when they opt for fertility treatment. I sincerely hope that in their quest to have a baby, they remain mindful of the major role that Nature plays in ultimately controlling conception. If they are able to do so, their journey will certainly be a less arduous one.

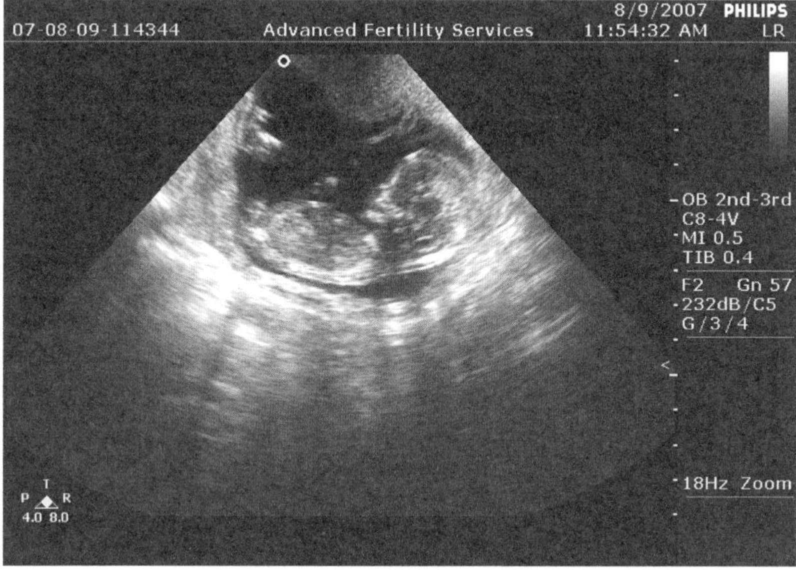

Fig. 1. ***A sonographic picture of a viable pregnancy***

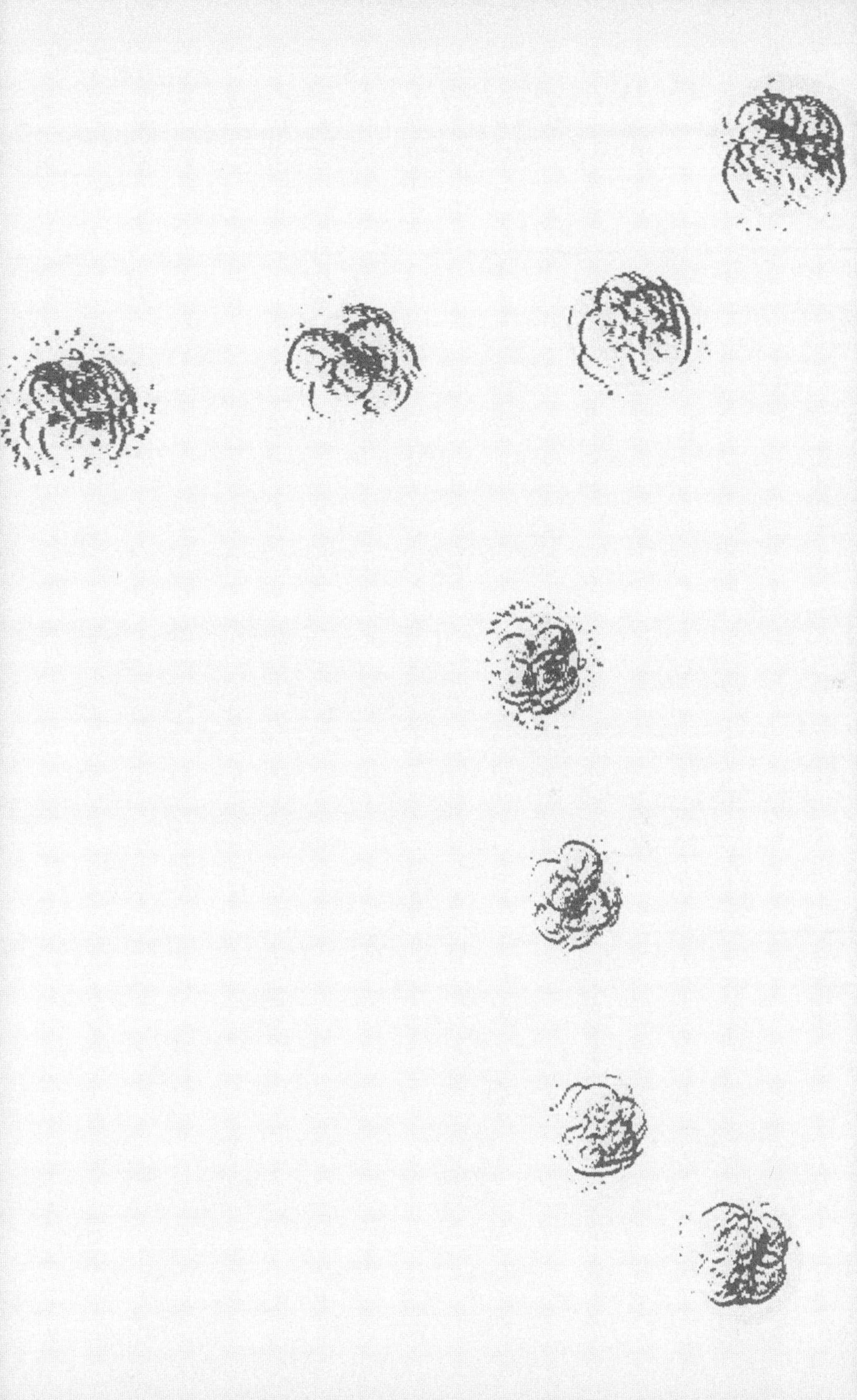

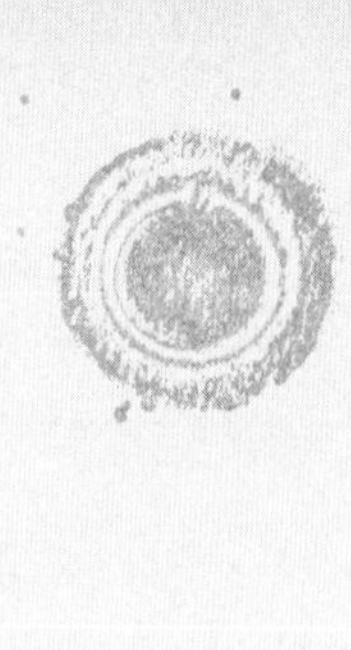
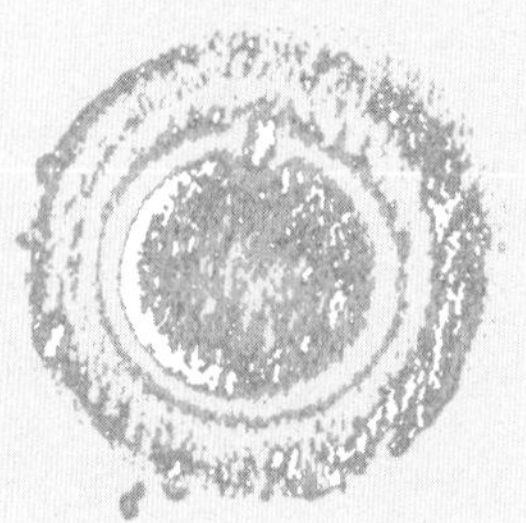
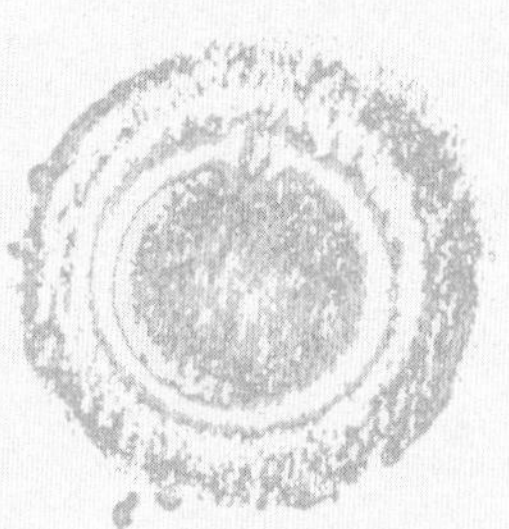
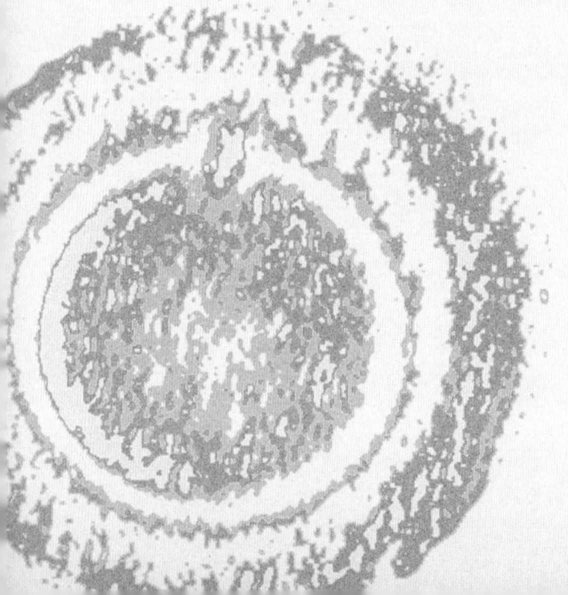

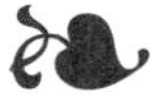

GLOSSARY

A

Acrosome: the package of enzymes at the tip of the sperm that help it penetrate the egg
Adenomyosis: the condition in which endometriosis exists in the muscular layer of the uterus
Adhesions: two separate surfaces, stuck to each other
Aneuploidy: a condition in which an embryo has too much or too little genetic material
Antagon: Fertility Drug
Antibody: a substance created by one's own immune system to fight off a "foreign" invader, like a bacteria or a virus
Antichlamydial antibodies: a substance created by the body to fight infection by the organism, chlamydia, which remains in the body and provides indication of a prior infection
Aspirate: the use of suction to remove fluid from a container or from somewhere in the body
Assisted hatching: a micromanipulation procedure in which the embryologist thins the zona pellucida of the embryo before it is transferred
Autoimmune disease: an illness caused by the body attacking its own tissues
Azoospermia: the condition in which a male's semen contains no sperm

B

Basal body temperature (BBT): body temperature at rest, immediately upon awakening. Charting a woman's daily BBT was a common method of determining if ovulation had occurred.
Blastocyst: an advanced embryo
Blastomere: one of the individual cells that make up an embryo.
Bravelle: Fertility Drug

C

Cetrotide: Fertility Drug
Chimeric embryo: an embryo that has two distinct cell populations originating from more than one zygote
Chlamydia: an infectious organism which may cause irreparable damage to the Fallopian tubes
Cilia: the hairs that line the inner Fallopian tubes
Clomiphene citrate: an oral fertility medication (brand names: Clomid, Serophone)
Co-culture: living cells that are added to the commercially-produced culture media used in IVF
Controlled Ovarian Hyperstimulation (COH): the use of fertility drugs to induce a woman's ovaries to produce multiple oocytes during a single cycle

Cryopreservation: the storage of live tissue, such as sperm or embryos, by freezing

Cul de sac: the area behind the uterus where mature eggs are released by the ovary (also known as the Pouch of Douglas)

Cumulus cells: the cells that surround a newly-released oocyte

D

Demerol: meperidine hydrochloride, a pain-relieving narcotic medication

Distal: farther

DNA: deoxyribonucleic acid, the molecules which make up an individual's unique genetic structure and which determine hereditary characteristics

E

Embryo: the initial stage of life, formed just after the egg has been fertilized by the sperm

Endometrial biopsy: a diagnostic fertility test in which a portion of the endometrium is removed from the uterus and examined by a pathologist

Endometriosis: the condition in which tissue microscopically similar to the uterine lining is found outside of the uterus, on the surfaces of the Fallopian tubes and ovaries

Endometrium: the tissue that lines the inside of the uterus

Epididymis: the tube-like portion of the male anatomy which extends from the testes. Sperm mature as they swim the length of the epididymis.

Epididymitis: inflammation of the epididymis

Estradiol: naturally-occurring estrogen

Estrogen: the basic female hormone

F

Falloposcope: an instrument that allows the doctor to look inside the Fallopian tubes

Follistim: an injectable fertility drug consisting of FSH

Fibroid: a benign tumor of the uterus

Fimbria: finger-like projections at the far ends of the Fallopian tubes

Follicle: the ovarian sac (or cyst) in which the oocyte develops

Follicle-stimulating hormone (FSH): the hormone that stimulates egg production

Follicular puncture: process by which mature follicles are removed from the ovary via a needle which is passed through the rear wall of the vagina

Follistim: Fertility Drug
Fragment: when parts of an embryo begin to break up

G

Genetic mosaicism: cases in which an embryo contains two or more cell populations that differ in genetic makeup and arise from a single zygote
Genetic mutation: an alteration in the nature of a gene
Gonadotropin: a hormone that acts directly on the ovary to stimulate the production of an egg (oocyte)
Gonal-F: Fertility Drug
Granulosa cells: cells that surround the oocyte

H

Hamster egg penetration test: a fertility test that evaluates the potential ability of a male's sperm to fertilize a human egg, it is rarely used today.
HCG: human chorionic gonadotropin, the early pregnancy hormone that, in injectable form, acts like LH, causing the final steps of egg development
Heparin: a blood thinner
Hydrosalpinx: a condition caused by a prior infection which causes the Fallopian tube to become filled with fluid
Hyperthyroidism: the condition in which the thyroid is overly active
Hypothalamus: a control center in the brain which governs ovulation by stimulating the pituitary gland
Hypothyroidism: the condition in which the thyroid gland is underactive
Hysterosalpingogram (HSG): dye-assisted x-ray of the uterus and Fallopian tubes

I

In vitro: out of the body
***In vitro* Fertilization:** procedure in which a woman's eggs are fertilized outside of her body and the resulting embryos are transferred back to her uterus
In vivo: in the body
Intracytoplasmic sperm injection (ICSI): the procedure in which a single sperm is injected into an egg to achieve fertilization
Intraperitoneal Insemination (IPI): a procedure in which processed sperm are injected through the rear wall of the vagina into the cul de sac at the time of ovulation
Intrauterine Insemination (IUI): a procedure which calls for processed sperm to be inserted into the top of the woman's uterus

IVIG: intravenous therapy with gamma globulin (pooled antibodies)

L

Laparoscopy: a surgical procedure in which a telescope is inserted through a small incision in the woman's abdomen for diagnostic and/or therapeutic purposes
Letrozle (Femara): Fertility Drug
Leukocyte: white blood cell
Leuvaris: Fertility Drug
Luteal phase defect: inadequate progesterone secretion during the postovulatory phase of a woman's menstrual cycle
Luteinized Unruptured Follicle (LUF) Syndrome: condition in which it appears that ovulation has occurred, but the egg is not actually released from the ovary
Luteinizing hormone (LH): the hormone which causes the final step of egg maturation

M

Meiosis: the process of reduction division, when the number of chromosomes contained in the egg reduces from 46 to 23
Menopur: Fertility Drug
Metaphase II: the name for the stage of egg development that occurs after the number of chromosomes has reduced from 46 to 23
Metrodin: an injectable fertility drug consisting of FSH, not currently being produced. Metrodin was equivalent to Fertinex, but needed to be administered intramuscularly rather than subcutaneously
Micromanipulate: to perform procedures on minuscule structures under the microscope
Microsurgical Epididymal Sperm Aspiration (MESA): a procedure to extract sperm from men with obstructions in their epididymal ducts
Monosomy: cases in which one of the twelve chromosome pairs tested in PGD is found to have only one strand
Morphology: shape
Morula: the embryonic stage which occurs 4 to 5 days after fertilization and is characterized by a mass of cells within the zona pellucida
Motility: movement
Mycoplasma: a bacteria-like organism sometimes found in the reproductive tract, that may (or may not) be related to infertility and miscarriage

O

Oocyte: developing egg

Ovarian Hyperstimulation Syndrome (OHSS): condition caused by fertility drugs, in which an unidentified substance causes the fluid component of blood to seep through the walls of the blood vessels into the patient's abdomen or chest cavities

Ovidrel: Fertility Drug

P

Patent: open

Pituitary gland: the gland responsible for production of the reproductive hormones FSH and LH

Polar body: the structure created during fertilization, which contains the extra chromosomal material eliminated by the developing oocyte or the embryo after it is fertilized

Polycystic Ovary Disease (PCO): condition in which the ovary contains numerous, small immature follicular (egg) cysts and may be associated with irregular periods, infertility and other symptoms. It is a genetic condition.

Polyspermy: condition in which an egg is fertilized by more than one sperm

Post-coital test (PCT): test of whether the male's sperm are able to reach and survive in the female's cervical mucus

Pouch of Douglas: the area behind the uterus where mature eggs are released by the ovary (also called the cul de sac)

Pregnyl: Fertility Drug

Preimplantation genetic diagnosis (PGD): a procedure that is employed to analyze certain aspects of the chromosomal content of individual embryos

Progesterone: the hormone produced during the second half of the menstrual cycle

Prolactin: the hormone responsible for causing milk secretion

Pronuclei: a mass of genetic material found inside an egg soon after entry of the sperm

Prostatitis: inflammation of the prostate gland

Proximal: near

R

Repronex: Fertility Drug

S

Seminal plasma: fluid in the ejaculate

Sonogram: an image created through ultrasound technology

Spindle mechanism: the mechanism on which the chromosomes of the egg and sperm are arranged for distribution during

the course of fertilization
Subcutaneous: below the skin
Superovulation: the process of using fertility drugs to induce the ovary to produce multiple mature follicles per month

T

Tamoxifen (Novaldex): Fertility Drug
Translocation: instances in which portions of matching chromosome strands are interchanged with each other
Testicular Extraction of Sperm (TESE): the process which calls for the surgical extraction of small pieces of the testicle for the purpose of harvesting sperm

V

Varicocele: a varicose vein in the scrotum
Velocity: speed

Z

Zona pellucida: the outermost layer surrounding the oocyte and, eventually, the embryo.